CW01668888

Ambulance Questions

Second Edition

APAP Education

Publishing the highest quality training manuals for Ambulance Personnel since 1995

First Edition 1997

Published by
APAP Education
Freepost BS8483
Shepton Mallet, Somerset, BA4 5XT

Compiled by
Stephen Clinton
Operational Paramedic Supervisor

Clinical Proofreaders
Tony Hayward
Clinical Operations Officer

Avril Hayward
Operational Paramedic Supervisor

Ieuan Williams
Paramedic

Additional Proofreading
Vicki Coumbe, Shaun Davies
Ambulance Technicians

ISBN: 978-0-9534972-3-2

Whilst every effort has been made to ensure the accuracy of this publication, it should only be used as a guide and is no substitute for proper training by recognised instructors. Where differences exist between this publication and local protocols, local protocols should always be adhered to.

Contents

Contents

\# Karen Simpson - Stockport Group.
07908700841
Please Return

Questions

Amendment Number 1

Please amend the following questions and answers in line with the changes in the European Resuscitation Guidelines:

163. The ratio of inflations to compressions in one man CPR is:
A) 30 to 2
B) 12 to 5
C) 2 to 30
D) 1 to 15

184. Which of the following is NOT correct when carrying out CPR?
A) Ratio of 2 compressions to 30 inflations
B) Ratio of 30 compressions to 2 inflations
C) Pulse check every 3 cycles
D) Carotid pulse check lasting 5-10 seconds

285. The ratio of compressions to inflations for two operators should be:
A) 5-1
B) 1-5
C) 30-2
D) 2-30

337. The ratio of ventilations to compressions for two operators on an adult patient is:
A) 1-5
B) 5-1
C) 1-30
D) 2-30

504. The ratio of compressions to inflations when carrying out CPR on a baby is 15-2.

724. The inflation to compression ratio in two man CPR is 30-2.

ANSWERS

Page	Question	Answer
91	163	C
92	184	A
93	285	C
93	337	D
96	504	True
100	724	False 2 man CPR has the ratio of 30 compressions to 2 inflation.

1. One of the side effects of atropine is:
A) Dry mouth
B) Bradycardia
C) Hypertension
D) All of the above

2. The fallopian tubes are approximately how long?
A) 10cm
B) 10mm
C) 100cm
D) 10 inches

3. Which of the following does NOT usually occur during pregnancy?
A) Increase in pulse pressure
B) PVCs on the ECG
C) Decrease in pulse pressure
D) Syncope

4. What is the name of the orifice that allows foetal blood to pass directly from the right atrium to the left?
A) Foramen magnum
B) Ductus venosus
C) Fenestra ovalis
D) Foramen ovale

5. Which of the following is considered to be a normal foetal presentation?
A) Left occipito anterior
B) First vertex
C) Right occipito anterior
D) All of the above

6. A respiratory assessment can be broken down into how many disciplines?
A) 3
B) 4
C) 5
D) 2

7. A palpable femoral pulse would suggest a systolic BP of more than:
A) 70mmHg
B) 80mmHg
C) 90mmHg
D) 60mmHg

8. Which of the following is the odd one out?
A) Inspection
B) Palpation
C) Pallor
D) Percussion

9. Cavitation can be as a result of:
A) Blunt trauma
B) Abrasion
C) Burns
D) Poisoning

10. For how long should a patient be pre-oxygenated prior to an intubation attempt?
A) 30 seconds
B) 30 minutes
C) 20 seconds
D) 2 minutes

11. A suitable diameter of ET tube for an adult female would be:
A) 8.5mm
B) 7.5mm
C) 6.5mm
D) 9.5mm

12. Which is the odd one out?
A) Acetylcholine
B) Noradrenaline
C) Serotonin
D) Ventolin

13. Which of the following is NOT a sign of fluid overload?
A) Distended neck veins
B) Tachycardia
C) Bradycardia
D) Dyspnoea

14. Which of the following describes VF?
A) Chaotic activity within the ventricular myocardium
B) Wide bizarre QRS complexes at a quickened rate
C) Complete ventricular standstill
D) Complete atrial standstill

15. Lignocaine is normally used for the treatment of,
A) Bradycardia
B) Ventricular ectopics
C) Atrial ectopics
D) Supraventricular tachycardia

16. What is the chemical name for aspirin?
A) Disprol
B) Anadin
C) Paracetamol
D) Acetylsalicylic acid

17. The absorption rate for a drug administered via the intravenous route is approximately,
A) 2-3 minutes
B) 15-30 minutes
C) 30-60 seconds
D) 15 minutes

18. The normal pacemaker of the heart is the,
A) Atrioventricular node
B) Sinoatrial node
C) Right bundle branch
D) Bundle of His

19. Which of the following is the correct conductivity pathway?
A) SA node - AV node - Bundle of His
B) AV node - SA node - Bundle of His
C) SA node - Bundle of His - AV node
D) Bundle of His - AV node - SA node

20. All ECG machines in use in Britain have a paper speed of,
A) 25mm per second
B) 25cm per second
C) 25mm per minute
D) 25cm per minute

21. The P wave represents,
A) Ventricular depolarisation
B) Ventricular refractory period
C) Atrial depolarisation
D) Atrial refractory period

22. The range of the normal QRS complex measures:
A) 0.08 - 0.12 seconds
B) 4.00 - 12.00 seconds
C) 0.12 - 2.00 seconds
D) 2.00 - 20.00 seconds

23. The term used to describe an abnormally slow heart rate is:
A) Tachycardia
B) Bradycardia
C) Tachypnoea
D) None of the above

24. Wenckebach phenomenon refers to which type of rhythm?
A) Sinus arrest
B) First degree heart block
C) Second degree heart block
D) Third degree heart block

25. Which of the following would be a suitable cannula size for rapid fluid administration in an adult patient?
A) 20g
B) 22g
C) 23g
D) 16g

26. Cells that support and protect neurones are called:
A) Axons
B) Neuroglia
C) Dendrites
D) None of the above

27. Which aspect of the nasal cavity houses the olfactory region?
A) Superior
B) Inferior
C) Lateral
D) Distal

28. How many pieces of cartilage make up the larynx?
A) 6
B) 7
C) 8
D) 9

29. The complete ring of cartilage situated at the inferior border of the larynx is the:
A) Corniculate
B) Arytenoid
C) Cricoid
D) Thyroid

30. The primary bronchi emanate from the trachea at the level of,
A) T1
B) T2
C) T4
D) T5

31. What percentage of oxygen is transported dissolved within blood plasma?
A) 3%
B) 97%
C) 7%
D) 23%

32. The centres which dictate the basic rate and depth of respiration are housed within the:
A) Cerebrum
B) Medulla oblongata
C) Cerebellum
D) Lungs

33. Which of the following is the odd one out?
A) Basophils
B) Eosinophils
C) Neutrophils
D) Thrombocytes

34. What percentage of plasma is water?
A) 81%
B) 95%
C) 91.5%
D) 81.5%

35. Which of the following blood groups is said to be the universal recipient?
A) O
B) A
C) B
D) AB

36. A capillary network directly connects:
A) Arteries to veins
B) Arterioles to venules
C) Arteries to arterioles
D) Veins to venules

37. The upper section of the uterus is called the:
A) Body
B) Fundus
C) Cervix
D) Womb

38. Which of the following is the odd one out?
A) Sensory
B) Motor
C) Afferent
D) Inherent

39. Which of the following has an effect on ventricular contraction?
A) Hydrogen ion pump
B) Sodium potassium pump
C) Bicarbonate ion pump
D) Potassium ion pump

40. The ability to conduct an impulse is brought about by the:
A) Hydrogen ion pump
B) Sodium potassium pump
C) Protein pump
D) Sodium hot pump

41. Which of the following is the odd one out?
A) Cerebrum
B) Cerebellum
C) Diencephalon
D) Pia mater

42. The cerebrum is divided by the:
A) Longitudinal fissure
B) Vermis
C) Cerebral cortex
D) Thalamus

43. The pons varolii lies:
A) Inferior to the medulla, superior to the mid brain
B) Lateral to the mid brain and the medulla
C) Inferior to the mid brain, superior to the medulla
D) Superior to the cerebrum

44. The medulla oblongata is approximately how long?
A) 2.5cm
B) 2.5 inches
C) 2.5mm
D) 5.5cm

45. The structure that controls hormone output is called:
A) Hypothalamus
B) Thalamus
C) Vasomotor centre
D) Cauda equina

46. The inner layer of the meninges is called the:
A) Pia mater
B) Arachnoid mater
C) Dura mater
D) Periosteum

47. The total amount of CSF in the average adult nervous system is:
A) 5-8 litres
B) 4-5 litres
C) 80-150ml
D) 180-250ml

48. In LVF the amount of blood within the system is,
A) Raised
B) Lowered
C) Unchanged
D) Compromised

49. Multifocal PVCs arise from:
A) Atria only
B) Anywhere within the ventricles
C) One specific area within the ventricles
D) None of the above

50. Which of the following has the fastest absorption rate?
A) Intravenous
B) Intracardiac
C) Sublingual
D) Intramuscular

51. Which of the following is the odd one out?
A) Aortic branch
B) Circumflex branch
C) Marginal branch
D) Posterior interventricular branch

52. What would be the appropriate drug for the treatment of anaphylaxis?
A) Atropine
B) Adrenaline
C) Lignocaine
D) Nubain

53. Sodium lactate solution is a:
A) Protein based solution
B) Crystalloid solution
C) Glucose solution
D) Blood derivative

54. In cases of burns shock develops following:
A) Damage to nerves
B) Infarction
C) Escape of plasma
D) Toxaemia

55. Which is the best position to transport a patient with a haemothorax?
A) Prone
B) Supine
C) Injured side uppermost
D) Injured side down

56. Which of the following describes Dextrose 50%?
A) Stimulates insulin production
B) Mobilises glycogen
C) Isotonic solution
D) None of the above

57. The ECG of a paediatric patient in cardiac arrest will usually exhibit:
A) Asystole
B) Ventricular fibrillation
C) EMD
D) Ventricular tachycardia

58. Which of the following is NOT a function of the spinal cord?
A) Relay sensory messages to the brain
B) Perform reflex arcs
C) Relay motor impulses from the brain
D) Receive and relay messages from cranial nerves

59. What would your initial treatment be of an MI patient?
A) Adrenaline
B) Aspirin
C) Oxygen
D) Paracetamol

60. Which of the following is NOT part of the management of a child suffering from epiglottitis?
A) Administer oxygen
B) Reassure parents and relatives
C) Transport calmly and quietly in the sitting position
D) Examine throat and aspirate

61. At what speed does standard ECG paper travel?
A) 25mm per second
B) 30mm per second
C) 40mm per second
D) 10mm per second

62. Which of the following is most likely to produce hypovolaemic shock?
A) Severe head injury
B) Spinal cord injury
C) Ruptured spleen
D) Pott's fracture

63. The preferred position for a conscious child with epiglottitis is:
A) Sitting upright and leaning forward
B) Fowler position
C) Supine
D) Prone

64. What sign would you expect to see in an over-infused patient?
A) Distended neck veins
B) Bradycardia
C) Choking sensation
D) All of the above

65. A buffer agent alters plasma pH from:
A) Alkaline to acid
B) Acid to alkaline
C) Alkaline to neutral
D) None of the above

66. Which of the following is NOT a crystalloid substance?
A) Hartmann's
B) Gelofusine
C) Dextrose solution
D) Dextrose 10%

67. Which drug does NOT increase pulse rate?
A) Adrenaline
B) Ventolin
C) Atropine
D) Lignocaine

68. Under normal circumstances intubation should take no longer than:
A) 5 seconds
B) 10 seconds
C) 15 seconds
D) 20 seconds

69. A patient's survival following a myocardial infarct depends on:
A) Length of time heart muscle was affected
B) Depth of muscle affected
C) How much muscle was affected
D) Position of muscle affected

70. On what type of patient would you use the Apgar scale?
A) Newborn infants
B) Cardiac patients
C) Adult burn patients
D) Diabetics

71. Which of the following is a side effect of Diazemuls?
A) Tachycardia
B) Hypertension
C) Sedation
D) Hyperventilation

72. Which of the following is an early sign of circulatory overload?
A) Renal shut down
B) Dyspnoea
C) Ankle oedema
D) Pain at the site of infusion

73. Ergometrine is administered to achieve:
A) A reduction in blood pressure
B) An increase in blood pressure
C) Contraction of the uterus
D) Relaxation of the uterus

74. The amount of air taken in one normal breath is known as:
A) Inspiratory reserve
B) Vital capacity
C) Dead air space
D) Tidal volume

75. Which of the following is NOT an indication of pre-eclampsia?
A) Hypertension
B) Oedema
C) Proteinuria
D) Hypotension

76. Which of the following best describes 3rd Degree AV Block?
A) Shortened P-R Interval
B) Lengthened P-R Interval
C) Disassociation of the P wave and the QRS complex
D) Disassociation of the T wave and the QRS complex

77. Which of the following is a predisposing factor of heart disease?
A) Hypertension
B) Cigarette smoking
C) Lack of exercise
D) All of the above

78. Epiglottitis usually affects children over the age of 4 years.

79. A 9.5mm intubation tube would be suitable for an adult male.

80. There are 12 pairs of cranial nerves.

81. All unconscious patients should be intubated.

82. An increase in blood pressure and a fast pulse are signs of head injury.

83. Glucagon is secreted by the kidneys.

84. The medulla oblongata contains the pneumotaxic area.

85. The abdominal thrust can be used on any age of patient to remove an obstruction from the airway.

86. Dead air space constitutes approximately 500ml.

87. Morphine is a respiratory stimulant.

88. Smaller air passages contain more cartilage.

89. Henry's law describes a gas's solubility.

90. Bradycardia is a sign of LVF.

91. Cervical and brain trauma can be associated with maxillofacial injuries.

92. CSF is produced in the sagittal sinus.

93. The smell of acetone on a patient's breath is indicative of hyperglycaemia.

94. The apneustic area is situated within the cerebrum.

95. The kidneys secrete prothrombin.

96. The amount of blood pumped from either the left or right ventricle in one minute is called the stroke volume.

97. The cardioacceleratory centre is stimulated by acetylcholine.

98. The atrial reflex is also called the Bainbridge reflex.

99. The vasomotor centre is situated in the medulla.

100. Blood viscosity will affect peripheral resistance.

101. Leukocytes will decrease when infection is present.

102. The peripheral nervous system can be divided into two sections.

103. The normal cardiac cycle takes 8.0 seconds.

104. The medulla oblongata is divided into 4 hemispheres.

105. A foetal heart functions differently to a postnatal heart.

106. IV fluid replacement is NOT indicated in the treatment of hypovolaemic shock.

107. The patient in ventricular fibrillation will usually be unconscious.

108. Nubain is a synthetic opioid.

109. Sodium bicarbonate can be given by the ET route.

110. Coronary perfusion takes place during diastole.

111. Afferent nerves carry impulses towards the brain.

112. Sodium and potassium are examples of cations.

113. The SA node is situated high in the right ventricle.

114. Antepartum haemorrhage occurs after birth.

115. Blood type AB negative can be given to a B negative recipient.

116. Stroke volume is the amount of blood ejected in one minute.

117. The 3 lead ECG is based on Einstein's triangle.

118. The normal firing rate of the SA node is 45-50 bpm.

119. The aVR lead on an ECG is placed on the left leg.

120. Vertical squares on an ECG represent amplitude.

121. QRS complexes represent depolarisation of the ventricles.

122. Sinus bradycardia usually has a rate greater than 80 beats per minute.

123. A crystalloid substance will seep out of the vascular space in approximately 20 minutes.

124. A consistently lengthened P-R interval indicates first degree AV block.

125. There are 3 grades of difficulty for patient intubation.

126. Any cell in the myocardium is capable of initiating an impulse.

127. Pneumonia is an inflammation of the lung.

128. Myelinated fibres within the brain are known as white matter.

129. A premature baby's heat regulation centre is not fully developed and its heat production may be inadequate.

130. The trachea is lined with ciliated mucous membrane.

131. Bronchioles directly terminate in the alveoli sacs.

132. Horizontal lines on ECG paper represent time.

133. Cerebral oedema will be increased if carbon dioxide levels are allowed to increase.

134. A straight blade on a laryngoscope makes intubation of children easier.

135. Cardiac tamponade could be the cause of EMD.

136. In atrial flutter the P wave is replaced by an F wave.

137. A ruptured ectopic pregnancy on its own will not give rise to shock.

138. Adrenaline is a synthetic substance.

139. Atropine is a sympathetic blocking agent.

140. Barbiturates depress the respiratory centre.

141. Atropine is the favoured drug in the treatment of ventricular tachycardia.

142. A side effect of GTN is a headache.

143. During the second trimester the maternal cardiac output is decreased by 20-30%.

144. 1st degree heart block is a life threatening arrhythmia.

145. A transverse lie will prevent a spontaneous delivery.

146. Hartmann's is a colloid solution.

147 The larynx houses the vocal cords.

148. Pregnant women are less prone to vaso-vagal attacks.

149. The term isotonic means that a solution is similar in concentration to blood.

150. Sodium bicarbonate is an acid solution.

151. Chest palpation is carried out with the use of a stethoscope.

152. Rales are caused by a build up of fluid in the lungs.

153. Blood group AB is considered to be the universal recipient.

154. Blood group O is known as the universal donor.

155. The foetal heart has an orifice within the atrial septum called the foramen magnum.

156. An example of a colloid solution would be Haemaccel.

157. A patient should be extubated at the end of the inspiratory phase.

158. A 7.5mm intubation tube should be cut to a length of 21cm.

159. Patients with short muscular necks tend to be easier to intubate.

160. The medulla oblongata is the youngest part of the brain.

161. Which of the following is NOT a digestive process?
A) Ingestion
B) Absorption
C) Perspiration
D) Defecation

162. A patient feeling faint should be,
A) Sat up and given cold water to drink
B) Sat up and given warm drinks to calm
C) Laid down, legs elevated
D) Laid down, head raised

163. The ratio of inflations to compressions in one man CPR is:
A) 15 to 2 30-2
B) 12 to 5
C) 2 to 15
D) 1 to 5

164. The main priority when dealing with maxillo-facial injuries is:
A) Blood loss
B) Airway obstruction
C) Deformity of facial bones
D) Shock

165. The pin index connection yoke on an Entonox set has:
A) 1 pin
B) 2 pins
C) 3 pins
D) 4 pins

166. Vitamin C can be found in which of the following?
A) Liver
B) Milk
C) Fresh fruit
D) Cereals

167. Which of the following is an indication for the use of Entonox?
A) Severe chest pain
B) Severe chest injury
C) Severe head injury
D) Severe mental illness

168. Which structure within the cell is responsible for carrying genes?
A) Plasma
B) Nucleus
C) Cytoplasm
D) Cell Membrane

169. What percentage of the body is made up of fluid?
A) 18%
B) 40%
C) 60%
D) 30%

170. Muscles are divided into how many main groups?
A) 4
B) 3
C) 2
D) 8

171. The pnemonic PEEP means,
A) Positive End Exit Pressure
B) Positive End Expiratory Pressure
C) Positive Exit Entrance Pressure
D) Pulse End Expiratory Pressure

172. How many bones make up the human skeleton?
A) 120
B) 220
C) 406
D) 206

173. An oxygen regulator,
A) Regulates the flow of oxygen to the patient's mask
B) Regulates moisture content of the oxygen
C) Reduces the cylinder pressure to a workable pressure of 60psi
D) Regulates how much oxygen the patient needs

174. Which of the following is the odd one out?
A) Humerus
B) Femur
C) Radius
D) Maxilla

175. Anterior refers to:
A) Towards the surface
B) Away from the midline
C) Towards the front of the body
D) None of the above

176. Which of the following structures are situated within the thoracic cavity?
A) Heart, lungs, oesophagus
B) Heart, stomach, duodenum
C) Lungs, trachea, kidneys
D) Heart, lungs, large intestines

177. How many parts is the pharynx usually divided into?
A) 1
B) 3
C) 2
D) 4

178. At what point do vessels enter and leave the lungs?
A) Cricoid
B) Carina
C) Hilum
D) Mediastinum

179. The normal pH of blood is:
A) 7.0
B) 4.7
C) 7.4
D) less than 7

180. How much oxygen does expired air contain?
A) 0.04%
B) 16%
C) 20%
D) 4%

181. The term for difficulty in breathing is:
A) Dyspnoea
B) Tachypnoea
C) Cyanosis
D) Hypoxia

182. Which of the following is a sign or symptom of compression?
A) Cold and clammy
B) Gradual onset
C) Quick feeble pulse
D) Pale

X B

183. The outer layer of the skin is called:
A) Epidermis
B) Dermis
C) Follicle
D) Subcutaneous

X Epidermis

184. Which of the following is NOT correct when carrying out CPR?
A) Ratio of 2 compressions to 15 inflations
B) Ratio of 15 compressions to 2 inflations
C) Pulse check every 3 cycles
D) Carotid pulse check lasting 5-10 seconds

185. Hollow spaces within the brain are known as:
A) Ventricles
B) Atria
C) Subdural spaces
D) Epidurals

186. The meninges cover the brain and spinal cord, what is the middle one called?
A) Arachnoid mater
B) Pia mater
C) Dura mater
D) Mia mater

our
Dura
Arachnoid
Pia
IW

187. The length of the average adult spinal cord is:
A) 16-18 inches
B) 20-24 inches
C) 36-42 inches
D) 10-13 inches

188. In an adult the spinal cord terminates at the level of:
A) L5
B) Between L4 & L5
C) Between L1 & L2
D) T5

X L1 L2

189. How many pairs of spinal nerves are there?
A) 33
B) 30
C) 31
D) 12

190. What is the approximate diameter of the adult spinal cord?
A) 1 inch
B) 1/2 inch
C) 1/4 inch
D) 2 inches

191. Which of the following is NOT a function of cerebrospinal fluid?
A) Support nervous tissue
B) Maintain a uniform pressure around the brain
C) Provide clotting of haemorrhage within the brain
D) Bathe brain cells and remove waste products

192. Which of the following is NOT a category of hazardous substance?
A) Chemical
B) Radioactive
C) Organic
D) Biological

193. Which patient condition is of most priority?
A) Fractured leg
B) Lacerated wound to the head
C) Absence of breathing
D) Severe shock

194. Apnoea refers to:
A) Low blood pressure
B) High blood pressure
C) Cardiac arrest
D) Cessation of breathing

195. When treating a patient with severe chest pain, which of the following actions is NOT correct?
A) Keep patient warm
B) Calm patient down
C) Walk the patient around
D) Get help immediately

196. On an infant, which one of the following is correct with regard the rule of nines?
A) Front Trunk - 18%
B) Arm - 18%
C) Head - 14%
D) Leg - 18%

197. Which of the following is the odd one out?
A) Radius bone
B) Ulna bone
C) Humerus bone
D) Femur bone

198. How many spinal vertebrae are there?
A) 31
B) 33
C) 35
D) 37

199. Where are blood cells produced?
A) Heart
B) Skin
C) Liver
D) Bone marrow

200. If your patient has an injury to just one eye you must:
A) Cover just the injured eye
B) Do not cover either eye
C) Cover both eyes
D) Tell the patient to blink

201. Which is the odd one out? The basic principles of first aid are:
A) Preserve life
B) Promote recovery
C) Promote public relations
D) Prevent deterioration

202. Which is the odd one out in the treatment of a burn?
A) Cool the burn
B) Dress the burn to stop infection
C) Apply cream to ease the pain
D) Treat for shock

203. Which of the following is the odd one out?
A) Ingestion
B) Absorption
C) Inhalation
D) Radiation

204. A D size Entonox cylinder contains:
A) 5,000 litres
B) 500 litres
C) 50 litres
D) 550 litres

205. An oropharyngeal airway should be measured:
A) From the patient's nose to the earlobe
B) From the corner of the patient's mouth to the earlobe
C) From the corner of the patient's mouth to the angle of the jaw
D) From earlobe to earlobe

206. When assessing the size of a burn using the rule of nines for an adult, which of the following is NOT correct?
A) Arm = 9%
B) Leg = 18%
C) Head = 9%
D) Back = 9%

207. How much oxygen does a D size cylinder hold?
A) 1360 litres
B) 340 litres
C) 2000 litres
D) 200 litres

208. Which of the following is NOT a sign of asthma?
A) Coughing
B) Inspiratory Wheeze
C) Dyspnoea
D) Expiratory Wheeze

209. When describing the rib cage which of the following is correct?
A) 7 true ribs - 3 false ribs - 2 floating ribs
B) 6 true ribs - 4 false ribs - 2 floating ribs
C) 7 true ribs - 3 false ribs - 1 floating rib
D) 6 true ribs - 4 false ribs - 1 floating rib

210. The largest part of the brain is called the:
A) Cerebrum
B) Cerebellum
C) Medulla
D) Brain stem

211. Which structure contains the cardiac centre?
A) Medulla
B) Mediastinum
C) Cerebellum
D) Cerebrum

212. How many layers make up the meninges?
A) 1
B) 2
C) 3
D) 4

213. Which of the following is NOT a cause of epilepsy?
A) Injury at birth
B) Mental illness
C) Brain injury
D) Genetic abnormality

214. The term for a bone extremity is:
A) Epiphysis
B) Periosteum
C) Diaphysis
D) None of the above

215. How many pairs of ribs make up the rib cage?
A) 18 pairs
B) 8 pairs
C) 10 pairs
D) 12 pairs

216. The adult human heart weighs approximately:
A) 4-6oz
B) 8-11oz
C) 10-20oz
D) 1-2 lb

217. If a fracture has been caused through trauma which of the following is the odd one out?
A) Spiral
B) Oblique
C) Pathological
D) Transverse

218. Which of the following is a cause of angina?
A) High blood pressure
B) Lack of exercise
C) Anxiety
D) All of the above

219. Which of the following groups of organs all lie within the abdominal cavity?
A) Gall bladder, liver and pancreas
B) Oesophagus, aorta and lungs
C) Pancreas, vena cava and lungs
D) Kidneys, spleen and heart

220. How many vertebrae are fused together to form the sacrum?
A) 4
B) 5
C) 6
D) 7

221. When describing the correct number of spinal vertebrae, which of the following is correct when considering from the superior aspect?
A) 7 - 12 - 5 - 5 - 4
B) 7 - 12 - 6 - 5 - 3
C) 7 - 12 - 5 - 6 - 4
D) 7 - 12 - 6 - 4 - 4

222. Which is the odd one out?
A) Maxilla
B) Zygoma
C) Sphenoidal
D) Lacrimal

223. Which is the odd one out?
A) Radius
B) Ulna
C) Humerus
D) Tibia

224. Which of the following is NOT a form of epilepsy?
A) Petit mal
B) Status epilepticus
C) Grand mal
D) Grand epilepticus

225. An increased urine output is called:
A) Polydypsia
B) Polyuria
C) Polybladder
D) Polyuremia

226. Which of the following is NOT a consequence of a head injury?
A) Concussion
B) Contre-coup
C) Contre-clap
D) Compression

227. Which of the following is NOT a sign or symptom of concussion?
A) Slow full pulse
B) Cold and clammy
C) Pale
D) Shallow rapid breathing

228. Which of the following is NOT a sign or symptom of hypoglycaemia?
A) Profuse sweating and pale
B) Normal to shallow respirations
C) Acetone breath
D) Normal temperature

229. The inner layer of the heart is called the:
A) Epicardium
B) Myocardium
C) Endocardium
D) Pericardium

230. The main artery supplying blood to the liver is:
A) Carotid artery
B) Hepatic artery
C) Gastric artery
D) Renal artery

231. Which of the following is NOT a complication of a burn?
A) Shock
B) Respiratory tract damage
C) Hypertension
D) Infection

232. The medical term for a swelling filled with blood is:
A) Haematoma
B) Hyphema
C) Haematuria
D) Haemorrhage

233. When taking a pulse on an infant, which point should be used?
A) Carotid
B) Subclavian
C) Brachial
D) Femoral

234. Which of the following will stimulate the nervous system?
A) Barbiturates
B) Amphetamines
C) Narcotics
D) Solvents

235. Barbiturate medicines are nervous system:
A) Stimulants
B) Depressants
C) Coordinators
D) Enhancers

236. Paracetamol is also known as:
A) Acetaminophen
B) Acetylcholine
C) Acetylsalicylic acid
D) Amphetamine

237. Which of the following is NOT a corrosive acid?
A) Sulphuric
B) Oxalic
C) Quick lime
D) Carbolic

238. Which of the following arteries supplies the large intestines?
A) Pulmonary arteries
B) Mesenteric arteries
C) Hepatic arteries
D) Renal arteries

239. Which is the odd one out?
A) Peritoneal ligaments
B) The omenta
C) The ovary
D) The mesentery

240. When referring to fractures which is the odd one out?
A) Comminuted
B) Compound
C) Simple
D) Difficult

241. The heart muscle is known as:
A) Pericardium
B) Myocardium
C) Endocardium
D) Epicardium

242. In excess of what percentage can a burn be considered major?
A) 10%
B) 20%
C) 30%
D) 40%

243. Which of the following is contraindicated in the administration of oxygen?
A) Cyanide poisoning
B) Carbon monoxide poisoning
C) Paraquat poisoning
D) Alcohol poisoning

244. A D sized oxygen cylinder will hold:
A) 330 litres of gas
B) 340 litres of gas
C) 350 litres of gas
D) 360 litres of gas

245. Entonox cylinders have a pin index on the neck comprising:
A) 1 pin
B) 2 pins
C) 3 pins
D) 4 pins

246. Oxygen is stored in cylinders charged to:
A) 1000psi
B) 1500psi
C) 2000psi
D) 2500psi

247. Which is NOT a sign of left ventricular failure?
A) Sweating
B) Distended neck veins
C) Tachycardia
D) Full bounding pulse

248. Angina pectoris is caused by:
A) Atherosclerosis
B) Arthritis
C) Arteriolitis
D) Arteriosis

249. Which is NOT a function of blood?
A) Carries oxygen to the tissues
B) Protects from infection
C) Carries carbon dioxide to the tissues
D) Carries nutrients to the tissues

250. Which is the odd one out?
A) Aorta
B) Carotid Artery
C) Femoral Artery
D) Pulmonary Artery

251. Tarsals of the ankle. Which does not exist?
A) Cuneiform medial
B) Cuneiform intermedial
C) Cuneiform inferior
D) Cuneiform lateral

252. Which of the following is NOT true with regard to hyperglycaemia?
A) Dry flushed skin
B) Fruity breath smell
C) Rapid onset
D) Fever and thirst

253. The abdominal cavity houses the:
A) Lungs
B) Heart
C) Oesophagus
D) Pancreas

254. ECT stands for:
A) Electrocardiac therapy
B) Electroconvulsive therapy
C) Electrocranial therapy
D) Electroconvulsive timescale

255. How many bones make up the vertebral column?
A) 31
B) 32
C) 33
D) 34

256. The type of fracture occurring in old age or as a result of disease is called:
A) Oblique
B) Pathological
C) Spiral
D) Greenstick

257. Which of the following are signs and symptoms of a fracture?
A) Pain and swelling
B) Deformity and haemorrhage
C) Shortening and crepitus
D) All of the above

258. Which of the following is an example of a hinge joint?
A) Knee
B) Hip
C) Ankle
D) Shoulder

259. Which of the following is correct? The word distal means:
A) A point nearer the point of origin
B) A point further from the point of origin
C) A point towards the front of the body
D) A point towards the back of the body

260. Which is the odd one out?
A) Right hypochondrium
B) Umbilical
C) Left lumbar
D) Right clavicular

261. Which is the odd one out?
A) Nucleus
B) Plasma membrane
C) Epithelial membrane
D) Protoplasm

262. Glands without ducts secrete:
A) Hormones
B) Enzymes
C) Plasma
D) Haemoglobin

263. The cranium is formed from how many bones?
A) 4
B) 6
C) 8
D) 2

264. The skeletal system is NOT responsible for:
A) Enabling movement
B) Protection of organs
C) Production of blood cells
D) The passing of nervous impulses

265. The fibrous membrane that surrounds bone is called:
A) Periosteum
B) Peritoneum
C) Cartilage
D) Peristalsis

266. The inferior boundary of the thoracic cavity is the:
A) Diaphragm
B) Thoracic vertebrae and spine
C) Ribs and intercostal muscles
D) Sternum and ribs

267. Physiology means the:
A) Way in which an organ functions
B) Structure and position of an organ
C) Way in which one organ joins another
D) Way in which blood vessels join into other organs

268. Genes are described as:
A) Hereditary factors
B) Plasma membranes
C) Cytoplasmic processes
D) Chemical inhibitors

269. Which of the following is NOT a vertex presentation?
A) Left-occipito anterior
B) Left-occipito posterior
C) Persistent mento-posterior
D) Frank's breech

270. Abortion is the termination of pregnancy before:
A) Week 20 of development
B) Week 24 of development
C) Week 28 of development
D) Week 32 of development

271. Pulmonary embolism refers to a blood clot lodged in an artery in the:
A) Lungs
B) Brain
C) Leg
D) Heart

272. Pneumothorax is described as being:
A) Blood in the pleural cavity
B) Air in the pleural cavity
C) Acid in the pleural cavity
D) Water in the pleural cavity

273. Atmospheric air contains:
A) 20% oxygen - 0.04% carbon dioxide
B) 16% oxygen - 0.4% carbon dioxide
C) 20% oxygen - 0.4% carbon dioxide
D) 16% oxygen - 0.04% carbon dioxide

274. During expiration:
A) Diaphragm and intercostal muscles relax
B) Diaphragm and intercostal muscles contract
C) Diaphragm lowers and intercostal muscles relax
D) Diaphragm lowers and intercostal muscles contract

275. The skin is NOT responsible for:
A) Protection
B) Immunity
C) Regulating body temperature
D) Muscle tone

276. Which of the following signs and symptoms occur in bronchitis?
A) Tachypnoea
B) Dyspnoea
C) Productive cough
D) All of the above

277. Which of the following is the odd one out?
A) Cytoplasm
B) Nucleus
C) Cell membrane
D) Myocardium

278. Which of the following is the odd one out?
A) Larynx
B) Trachea
C) Oesophagus
D) Bronchi

279. Which of the following statements is true about the trachea?
A) It is approximately 14mm long
B) The D shaped cartilages open at the front
C) The C shaped cartilages open at the back
D) It is continuous with the oesophagus

280. The lining of the lungs is called the:
A) Pleura
B) Pericardium
C) Periosteum
D) Pericomo

281. When air passes through the alveoli wall, the process is called:
A) Osmosis
B) Diffusion
C) Respiration
D) Expiration

282. The respiratory centre is situated in the:
A) Cerebral cortex
B) Lungs
C) Larynx
D) Medulla oblongata

283. A patient who is unconsciou and has no other injuries should be placed in the:
A) Prone position
B) Recovery position
C) Supine position
D) Sitting position

284. When carrying out cardiac compressions on an adult you should attempt how many compressions per minute?
A) 50-60
B) 40-50
C) 60-70
D) 80-100

285. The ratio of compressions to inflations for two operators should be:
A) 5-1
B) 1-5
C) 15-2
D) 2-15

286. Which of the following is the odd one out?
A) Temporal
B) Frontal
C) Ethmoid
D) Mandible

287 The term “respiratory arrest” means:
A) Absence of breathing
B) Extreme difficulty in breathing
C) Absence of breathing and pulse
D) None of the above

288 Vital lung capacity is inspiratory reserve and:
A) Tidal volume and residual air
B) Tidal volume and expiratory reserve
C) Tidal volume
D) Minute volume

289 In asthma, the patient will:
A) Have difficulty exhaling
B) Have difficulty breathing while sitting up
C) Breathe easier lying down
D) Have none of the above

290 The brain is said to shrink in old age. By how much?
A) 5%
B) 10%
C) 15%
D) 29%

291 In the foetal circulation the pulmonary trunk is directly joined to the aorta by:
A) Ductus arteriosus
B) Ductus aorta
C) Ductus artery
D) Ductus venosus

292 The third stage of labour is the:
A) Stage in which the placenta is delivered
B) Actual birth of the baby
C) “Breaking of the waters”
D) Point at which crowning is seen

293 Antepartum haemorrhage occurs:
A) After month 4 of pregnancy but before stage 2 of labour
B) After month 5 of pregnancy but before stage 1 of labour
C) After month 6 of pregnancy but before stage 2 of labour
D) After month 4 of pregnancy but before stage 3 of labour

294. Primary postpartum haemorrhage is excessive bleeding up to how many hours after birth?
A) 18
B) 24
C) 27
D) 28

295. Which of the following is NOT a sign or symptom of Parkinson's disease?
A) Muscle tremor
B) Loss of coordination of the feet only
C) Muscle rigidity
D) Expressionless face

296. Which of the following is the odd one out?
A) Physical abuse
B) Sexual abuse
C) Perversion
D) Mental cruelty

297. The transformation of tissue into bone is called:
A) Organisation
B) Ossification
C) Haemolisis
D) Cancellation

298. Which of the following is the odd one out?
A) Head and neck tilt
B) Fowlor position
C) Recovery position
D) Back slaps

299. Which of the following is NOT a recognised precaution against infection?
A) Always wear rubber gloves
B) Thoroughly clean equipment after use
C) Wear a face mask
D) Use barrier cream

300. An F size oxygen cylinder contains:
A) 1360 litres charged to 1500psi
B) 1360 litres charged to 2000psi
C) 136 litres charged 1500psi
D) 136 litres charged to 2000psi

301. How many lobes are there in the right lung?
A) 1
B) 2
C) 3
D) 4

302. The trachea consists of which sort of lining?
A) Ciliated
B) Squamous
C) Synovial
D) Serous

303. The division between the lungs is called the:
A) Septum
B) Diaphragm
C) Mediastinum
D) Intercostal space

304. Orthopnoea means difficulty in breathing when:
A) Exercising
B) Lying down
C) At high altitude
D) Suffering chest pain

305. Which of the following describes the pleura?
A) Serous membrane
B) Mucous membrane
C) Fibrous membrane
D) Synovial membrane

306. The normal breathing rate of an adult is:
A) 8-12 per minute
B) 24-28 per minute
C) 16-20 per minute
D) 19-25 per minute

307. Which of the following structures contains no cartilage?
A) Trachea
B) Larynx
C) Bronchioles
D) Bronchi

308. Which of the following cartilages protects the trachea during the act of swallowing?
A) Cricoid
B) Thyroid
C) Epiglottis
D) Glottis

309. Asthma is described as spasm of the:
A) Bronchial cartilage
B) Bronchial smooth muscle
C) Larynx
D) Vocal cords

310. The bifurcation of the trachea is called the:
A) Web
B) Carina
C) Fissure
D) Guard

311. In which of the following cavities do you find the respiratory centre?
A) Thoracic
B) Abdominal
C) Cranial
D) Pelvic

312. The most common indirect method of contracting an infection is:
A) Airborne
B) Handling a patient's clothing
C) Contact with faeces or urine
D) Using the toilet after an infected patient

313. Infection can enter the body in one of several different ways. Which of the following is the odd one out?
A) Inhalation
B) Ingestion
C) Sexual transmission
D) Radiation

314. Which of the following is NOT a sign of cardiac arrest?
A) No pulse
B) No breathing
C) Pinpoint pupils
D) Blueness of the face

315. Which is the odd one out?
A) Smallpox
B) Lassa Fever
C) Rabies
D) Whooping Cough

316. Jaundice is usually a sign of:
A) COAD
B) Hepatic problems
C) Cardiomyopathy
D) Duodenal ulcer

317. Which of the following is the odd one out?
A) Anthrax
B) Cholera
C) Dysentry
D) Influenza

318. A full thickness burn affects:
A) Only the dermis
B) Only the epidermis
C) The layers of skin and underlying tissues
D) Only the dermis and epidermis

319. Which of the following is NOT a predisposing factor of a burn?
A) Fires as a result of road traffic accidents
B) Fireworks
C) Molten metal injuries associated with industry
D) Time of day the burn occurred

320. Which of the following is NOT correct concerning a closed fracture?
A) Pain
B) Swelling
C) Crepitus
D) Lengthening

321. The average tidal volume of a male adult is:
A) 200ml
B) 300ml
C) 400ml
D) 500ml

322. With regard to the Glasgow Coma Scale, which is the odd one out?
A) Motor response
B) Pupillary response
C) Eye response
D) Verbal response

323. With regard to the rule of nines for an adult patient, which of the following is NOT correct?
A) Hand = 1%
B) Whole leg = 18%
C) Whole arm = 18%
D) Head = 9%

324. The respiratory system is NOT responsible for:
A) Taking oxygen into the body
B) Regulating acid base balance of the blood
C) Protection from infection
D) Expelling carbon dioxide from the body

325. Which is the odd one out?
A) Petit mal
B) Status epilepticus
C) Gene mal
D) Grand mal

326. Which is the odd one out? CSF:
A) Is responsible for maintaining uniform pressure around nerve tissue
B) Is responsible for supplying nerve tissue with nutrients
C) Is responsible for protection against trauma
D) Acts as a neurotransmitter

327. The pons varolii houses which of the following centres?
A) Cardiac centre
B) Vasomotor centre
C) Reticular formation
D) Pneumotaxic area

328. The hypothalamus is NOT responsible for which of the following?
A) Regulation of hunger and food intake
B) Regulation of body temperature
C) Control of voluntary skeletal muscle
D) Rage and aggression

329. CSF fills which of the following spaces?
A) Subarachnoid space
B) Subdural space
C) Subpia space
D) Dural-pia space

330. The mid brain:
A) Acts as a relay station between different parts of the brain
B) Contains the respiratory rhythmacity centre
C) Regulates bodily water intake and thirst
D) Registers the senses of smell, taste and hearing

331. The cerebellum is divided into two hemispheres by the:
A) Vermis
B) Wermis
C) Tardis
D) Cortex

332. The three phases of respiration are:
A) Expiration, pause, inspiration
B) Inspiration, expiration, pause
C) Expiration, inspiration, pause
D) Pause, inspiration, expiration

333. Neuroglia is NOT:
A) Responsible for support and protection of nerve cells
B) Responsible for shaping nerve cells
C) Responsible for the production of myelin sheath
D) Formed from schwann cells

334. Which of the following is NOT a sign or symptom of asphyxia?
A) Anxiety
B) Congestion of neck veins
C) Cyanosis
D) Dehydration

335. Which is the odd one out with regard to lifting technique?
A) Back straight
B) Stand as close as possible to the object to be lifted
C) Chin tucked in
D) Stand with feet apart

336. There are three main subjects to be considered when making a patient assessment, which is the odd one out?
A) History
B) Airway
C) Signs
D) Symptoms

337. The ratio of ventilations to compressions for two operators on an adult patient is:
A) 1-5
B) 5-1
C) 1-15
D) 2-15

338. Which officer does NOT have a designated role at the scene of a major incident?
A) Incident Officer
B) Liaison Officer
C) Chief Ambulance Officer
D) Parking Officer

339. A major incident is defined as requiring special arrangements due to:
A) Location and number of casualties
B) Types of chemicals involved
C) Types of injuries to patients
D) Number of ambulance personnel required

340. Which is the odd one out?
A) Obeys commands
B) Spontaneous
C) Open to speech
D) Open to pain

341. Which is the odd one out?
A) Pain
B) Tingling
C) Skin colour
D) Memory loss

342. Which is the odd one out?
A) Haemorrhage
B) Crepitus
C) Nausea
D) Vomiting

343. Which of the following defines the functions of the respiratory system?
A) To provide oxygen for the tissues and remove carbon dioxide
B) To maintain blood pressure
C) To provide nutrients to the tissues
D) To maintain enzyme balance within the body

344. Bronchitic sputum is usually thick:
A) Greenish yellow
B) Blackish green
C) Blackish orange
D) Greenish brown

345. Multipolar neurones are found mainly within the:
A) Ganglia of cranial nerves
B) Retina of the eye
C) Brain and spinal cord
D) Olfactory region

346. Which of the following is the odd one out?
A) Thoracic
B) Lumbar
C) Abdominal
D) Cranial

347. A patient relying on hypoxic drive is stimulated to breathe by:
A) Low levels of carbon dioxide
B) High levels of carbon dioxide
C) Low levels of oxygen
D) High levels of oxygen

348. Pneumonia is usually as a result of:
A) Infection
B) Exertion
C) Allergy
D) Stress

349. Which type of shock occurs as a result of haemorrhage?
A) Anaphylactic
B) Cardiogenic
C) Neurogenic
D) Hypovolaemic

350. Which of the following is NOT usually a sign of shock?
A) Hypotension
B) Hypertension
C) Tachycardia
D) Pallor

351. Croup usually affects which age group?
A) 5-10 years
B) 6 months to 4 years
C) 12 years onwards
D) 2-4 months

352. Which of the following responses does not fall into the motor response category of the Glasgow Coma Scale?
A) Obeys commands
B) Extensor response
C) Eye movement
D) No response

353. Which of the following is NOT a sign of acute asthma?
A) Thick yellow-green sputum
B) Dyspnoea
C) Cyanosis
D) Wheezing

354. Which of the following is NOT a synovial joint?
A) Ball and socket
B) Slightly moveable
C) Double hinge
D) Pivot

355. Which of the following is NOT a synovial joint?
A) Elbow
B) Symphysis pubis
C) Lower jaw
D) Shoulder

356. Colic pain can be described as:
A) Intermittent
B) Continuous
C) Localised
D) Referred

357. Which is the odd one out?
A) Femur
B) Tibia
C) Fibula
D) Knee Cap

358. Which of the following statements is true of epithelial tissue?
A) Connects all other tissue together
B) Receives and transmits electrical stimuli
C) Initiates movement
D) Provides coverings and linings for organs

359. Which of the following is the odd one out?
A) Signs
B) Symptoms
C) History
D) Diagnosis

360. Which of the following is NOT a symptom?
A) Swelling
B) Nausea
C) Pain
D) Dizziness

361. When checking the pulse you should aim to ascertain:
A) The patient's colour
B) Rate, rhythm and strength
C) Level of consciousness
D) None of the above

362. The Glasgow Coma Score is divided into how many categories?
A) 1
B) 2
C) 3
D) 4

363. If the patient has no pulse then you should:
A) Turn the patient into the recovery position
B) Treat any haemorrhage
C) Instigate resuscitation
D) Check the Glasgow Coma Score

364. When checking the patient's breathing you would look at:
A) Rate and depth
B) Rhythm and sound
C) Odour
D) All of the above

365. In the average adult the heart pumps approximately how many beats per minute?
A) 120
B) 75
C) 175
D) 45

366. Which of the following is a sign of an MI?
A) Dyspnoea
B) Nausea
C) Chest pain
D) All of the above

367. How many teeth does a healthy adult have?
A) 30
B) 26
C) 34
D) 32

368. When arriving at the scene of an accident you must:
A) Check for haemorrhage
B) Check for fractures
C) Check for danger
D) Call for the police

369. Which of the following is NOT one of the principles of ambulance aid?
A) Preserve life
B) Promote recovery
C) Provide rapid journey to hospital
D) Prevent deterioration

370. Which of the following is correct with regard to the Glasgow Coma Scale?
A) There are 5 levels of eye response
B) There are 6 levels of verbal response
C) There are 5 levels of motor response
D) None of the above

371. Which of the following is NOT a sign of a fracture?
A) Pain
B) Abnormal movement
C) Deformity
D) Crepitus

372. Which of the following is NOT a complication of a pelvic fracture?
A) Damage to the bladder
B) Damage to major blood vessels
C) Damage to the spinal cord
D) Damage to the urethra

373. Which of the following is the odd one out?
A) Pharynx
B) Larynx
C) Oesophagus
D) Buccal Cavity

374. The most common cause of mental handicap is:
A) Padgett's disease
B) Cerebral palsy
C) Downs syndrome
D) Spina bifida

375. What must you NOT do when dealing with the deaf?
A) Speak clearly and slowly
B) Over exaggerate lip movements
C) Use gestures to make yourself clear
D) Raise voice slightly

376. A hypoglycaemic attack will occur:
A) Over several days
B) Over many weeks
C) Suddenly
D) None of the above

377. The serous membrane lining the abdomen is:
A) Periseal
B) Peritoneum
C) Peristaltic
D) Periosteum

378. The first stage of labour usually lasts approximately:
A) 12-14 hours
B) Over 24 hours
C) Over 48 hours
D) Less than 2 hours

379. When full the bladder normally holds:
A) 200ml
B) 500ml
C) 300ml
D) 600ml

380. With regard to the Glasgow Coma Score, withdraws from pain scores:
A) 5
B) 4
C) 3
D) 2

381. A low level of oxygen in the tissues is called:
A) Hypoxia
B) Carboxia
C) Hypoxaemia
D) Anaemia

382. The epiglottis is found:
A) At the top of the pharynx
B) At the bottom of the pharynx
C) Under the pharynx
D) At the base of the nasopharynx

383. Bile from the liver enters the digestive system at the:
A) Stomach
B) Jejunum
C) Duodenum
D) Small intestine

384. The axis bone can be found in the:
A) Ear
B) Spine
C) Ankle
D) Wrist

385. The ischium is part of the:
A) Small intestine
B) Cranium
C) Pelvis
D) Brain

386. Which is the odd one out?
A) Cervical collar
B) RED
C) Orthopaedic stretcher
D) Aspirator

387. The outer layer of the blood vessel is called the:
A) Tunica media
B) Tunica intima
C) Tunica adventitia
D) Tunica in brine

388. Dysarthia means:
A) Weakness of lower limb muscles
B) Incontinence
C) General mental confusion
D) Weakness of muscles of speech

389. The skin is responsible for which of the following?
A) Regulating body temperature
B) Protection
C) Immunity
D) All of the above

390. Which of the following is the odd one out?
A) Radial
B) Abdominal
C) Carotid
D) Brachial

391. The amount of atmospheric air that flows in and out with every normal breath is termed:
A) Stroke volume
B) Minute volume
C) Tidal volume
D) None of the above

392. Gaseous exchange between the alveoli and the surrounding capillaries takes place by:
A) Osmosis
B) Diffusion
C) Systolic BP
D) Respiration

393. What is the approximate length of the trachea?
A) 12cm
B) 4.5cm
C) 12 inches
D) 2.5cm

394. Which of the following functions of the nasal cavity is the odd one out?
A) Filtering
B) Cooling
C) Moistening
D) Warming

395. Which of the following is false? Poisons can be:
A) Ingested into the body
B) Injected into the body
C) Inhaled into the body
D) Projected into the body

396. How many stages can labour be divided into?
A) 4
B) 3
C) 2
D) 1

397. Which of the following treatments is false with regard to corrosive poisoning?
A) Seek medical attention
B) Turn unconscious patients into recovery position
C) Maintain an open airway
D) If conscious try to induce vomiting

398. Which of the following is the inner most layer of the heart?
A) Myocardium
B) Endocardium
C) Epicardium
D) Pericardium

399. Which of the following is NOT a sign of hypoglycaemia?
A) Fruity breath smell
B) Hunger
C) Headache
D) Pale skin

400. A grand mal seizure has how many stages?
A) 1
B) 2
C) 3
D) 4

401. When assessing a burn on an infant, the whole of one arm would be equal to:
A) 9%
B) 18%
C) 14%
D) 10%

402. Which of the following is the odd one out with regard to the treatment of burns?
A) Cool the burn
B) Safety to yourself
C) Administration of cups of sweet tea
D) Ensure the patient is breathing

403. Which of the following is NOT a sign of hypothermia?
A) Cold, pale, dry skin
B) Slow, weak pulse
C) Fast, bounding pulse
D) Slow, shallow breathing

404. Which of the following is NOT a natural mechanism to prevent bodily heat loss?
A) Constriction of peripheral blood vessels
B) Erection of body hairs
C) Increased breathing rate
D) Shivering

405. Which of the following is the odd one out?
A) Sulphuric acid
B) Quick lime
C) Phenol
D) Acetic acid

406. A pulse point is:
A) Anywhere there is an artery
B) Where an artery crosses a vein
C) Where a vein crosses a bone
D) Where an artery crosses a bone

407. The aorta is responsible for passing blood from:
A) The heart to the body
B) The heart to the lungs
C) The lungs to the heart
D) The body to the heart

408. What is the term used to describe inadequate perfusion of the myocardium?
A) Anoxia
B) Thrombosis
C) Hypoxia
D) Ischaemia

409. Which of the following is the odd one out?
A) SA node
B) AV node
C) Bundle of His
D) Interventricular septum

410. In hypothermia which of the following is correct?
A) Breathing rate will slow down
B) Breathing rate will speed up
C) The body will sweat
D) All of the above

411. Which of the following is NOT included in the treatment of a patient with spinal injury?
A) Maintain head and neck in neutral position
B) Reassure patient and encourage to keep still
C) Give a hot sweet drink
D) Keep the patient warm

412. Which of the following is the term for blood in the pleural cavity?
A) Haemothorax
B) Pneumothorax
C) Pulmonary embolism
D) Emphysema

413. Which of the following is true with regard to an incised wound?
A) Results from ripping or snagging of the tissues by metal or similar
B) A superficial wound resulting in the upper layers of skin being scraped off
C) Caused by rupture of the underlying vessels from a blow or blunt force
D) A clean cut made by a sharp edge or knife

414. The average adult blood volume is:
A) 3-4 litres
B) 8-9 litres
C) 1-2 litres
D) 5-6 litres

415. When a coronary artery becomes completely blocked, which of the following conditions occur?
A) Left ventricular failure
B) Angina pectoris
C) Myocardial infarction
D) Congestive heart failure

416. Which of the following is NOT a sign or symptom of shock?
A) Slow pulse
B) Nausea
C) Cold, clammy skin
D) Weakness

417. The middle layer of the heart is called:
A) Pericardium
B) Myocardium
C) Epicardium
D) Endocardium

418. The right atrium and ventricle are connected by which valve?
A) Bicuspid
B) Tricuspid
C) Aortic
D) Systemic

419. The bones forming the fingers are called:
A) Metacarpals and phalanges
B) Metatarsals and phalanges
C) Tarsals and phalanges
D) Humerus and carpals

420. Cells responsible for the carriage of haemoglobin are called:
A) Leukocytes
B) Erythrocytes
C) Phagocytes
D) Lymphocytes

421. At which point is the myocardium thickest?
A) Base
B) Left atrium
C) Right ventricle
D) Left ventricle

422. Blood leaving the heart from the left ventricle passes to the:
A) Inferior vena cava
B) Superior vena cava
C) Pulmonary artery
D) Aorta

423. Which of the following is NOT a component of a neurone?
A) Dendrite
B) Cell body
C) Axon
D) Gland

424. The largest part of the brain is the:
A) Medulla oblongata
B) Pons varolii
C) Cerebrum
D) Cerebellum

425. The cerebellum controls:
A) Muscle coordination
B) Muscle tone
C) Posture and balance
D) All of the above

426. Which of the following is NOT a sign of compression injury to the brain?
A) Headache
B) Fast pulse
C) Unequal pupils
D) Flushed complexion

427. The inner layer of the meninges surrounding the brain is called the:
A) Pia mater
B) Arachnoid mater
C) Dura mater
D) Cerebral cortex

428. The medulla oblongata regulates:
A) Muscle tone
B) Heart rate
C) ESP
D) Posture and balance

429. Which of the following is NOT a treatment for infantile convulsions?
A) Monitor the airway
B) Keep the child warm
C) Remove clothing
D) Seek medical attention as a precaution

430. The fluid surrounding the brain and spinal cord is called:
A) Synaptic fluid
B) Plasma
C) Cerebrospinal fluid
D) Synovial fluid

431. Section 3 of the Mental Health Act 1983 allows:
A) Emergency admission for 72 hours for assessment
B) Patient to admit themselves for unspecified time
C) Admission for minimum of 28 days for assessment
D) Admission for 6 months for treatment

432. Which of the following vessels supplies the liver with oxygenated blood?
A) Hepatic vein
B) Aorta
C) Hepatic artery
D) Mesenteric artery

433. Which part of a neurone is responsible for conducting the impulse towards the cell body?
A) Axon
B) Dendrite
C) Terminal arborisation
D) Medullary sheath

434. Which of the following is NOT found on a hazchem panel?
A) United Nations code number
B) 24 hour manufacturer's telephone number
C) Driver's telephone number
D) Hazard diamond appropriate to the substance

435. Which of the following is NOT a category 1 infectious disease?
A) Influenza
B) Scabies
C) Leprosy
D) Chicken pox

436. Which of the following means that a disease is always present in an area?
A) Sporadic
B) Epidemic
C) Pandemic
D) Endemic

437. A premature baby weighs less than:
A) 5kg
B) 2.5kg
C) 4lb
D) 2.5lb

438. When a patient is in labour, admission to hospital is advised when contractions occur every:
A) 20 minutes
B) 10 minutes
C) 25 minutes
D) 30 minutes

439. Which of the following is NOT a sign of cardiac arrest?
A) Unconsciousness
B) Equally contracted pupils
C) Absence of a carotid pulse
D) Cyanosis / grey colour

440. Which of the following is NOT a sign or symptom of shock?
A) Increased pulse rate
B) Increased blood pressure
C) Thirst
D) Nausea

441. The normal blood volume of a 1-2 year old is:
A) 0.5 litres
B) 0.7 litres
C) 1.0 litres
D) 1.5 litres

442. What % of blood volume is fluid?
A) 35%
B) 45%
C) 55%
D) 65%

443. The pericardium consists of an outer layer of:
A) Synovial membrane
B) Serious membrane
C) Synaptic membrane
D) Serous membrane

444. If an eye is injured by some foreign object embedded in it, should you:
A) Cover the affected eye with a sterile pad
B) Cover both eyes with sterile pads
C) Apply direct pressure to the eye
D) Leave well alone until hospitalisation

445. The AIDS virus can be transmitted by which of the following means?
A) Contact with an infected person's saliva
B) Contact with an infected person's blood
C) Contact with an infected person's clothing
D) Contact with an infected person's eating utensils

446. Blood loss in primary postpartum haemorrhage should not exceed:
A) 300ml
B) 400ml
C) 500ml
D) 600ml

447. The outer surface of the cerebrum is called:
A) Corpus
B) Cortex
C) Callosum
D) Pons varolii

448. Which of the following stimuli is NOT registered by the thalamus?
A) Cold
B) Sound
C) Pain
D) Heat

449. Which of the following will cause the pupils to constrict?
A) Severe bleeding
B) Intracranial pressure
C) Morphia poisoning
D) Death

450. The nerve controlling the diaphragm is called the:
A) Vagus
B) Phrenic
C) Glossopharyngeal
D) Maxilla

451. How many tarsals are there in the foot?
A) 6
B) 8
C) 7
D) 14

452. The lowest Glasgow Coma Score is:
A) 0
B) 3
C) 5
D) 15

453. A blood pressure taken at the height of ventricular contraction is called which value?
A) Diastolic
B) Systolic
C) Pulse pressure
D) None of the above

454. The Revised Trauma Score takes into account:
A) Pulse pressure - GCS - Skin colour
B) Respiratory rate - BP - GCS
C) Respiratory rate - BP - Respiratory depth
D) BP - Pulse - Respiratory rate

455. The best possible Glasgow Coma Score is:
A) 15
B) 20
C) 5
D) 10

456. Which of the following does NOT constitute part of the primary survey?
A) Airway
B) Circulation
C) Pupillary reaction
D) Level of consciousness

457. Which of the following is the odd one out?
A) Haemorrhage
B) Swelling
C) Deformity
D) Dizziness

458. 60% of body weight is fluid, what % is found inside the cells?
A) 30%
B) 55%
C) 70%
D) 40%

459. The length of a premature baby is less than:
A) 50 cm
B) 17 cm
C) 17 inches
D) 20 inches

460. Which of the following is NOT a sign or symptom of a CVA?
A) Pulse - slow and full
B) Pupils - unequal, dilated on affected side
C) Skin - pale and clammy
D) Hemiplegia

461. Which of the following is NOT a common cause of mental illness?
A) Anxiety
B) Depression
C) Hypotension
D) Obsessions

462. Haemodialysis patients are prone to suddenly becoming:
A) Hypertensive
B) Hypotensive
C) Hypothermic
D) Hypochondriac

463. Convulsions associated with pregnancy are called:
A) Pre-eclampsia
B) Elclampsia
C) Post-clampsia
D) Eclampsia

464. What level of oxygen is required in the treatment of suspected cardiac chest pain?
A) 3-4 litres per minute
B) 6-8 litres per minute
C) 2-4 litres per minute
D) 10+ litres per minute

465. Difficult, laboured breathing is known as:
A) Orthopnoea
B) Dyspnoea
C) Apnoea
D) Difpnoea

466. Which of the following is most likely to result in oedema of the lower extremities?
A) Myocardial infarct
B) Congestive heart failure
C) Angina pectoris
D) Cardiac arrest

467. A pulse point is:
A) Anywhere there is an artery
B) Where an artery crosses a bone
C) Where a vein crosses a bone
D) Where an artery crosses a vein

468. In the unconscious patient the most important thing to assess is:
A) Presence of a head injury
B) Check ears for fluid loss
C) Airway clear of obstructions
D) Presence of major haemorrhage

469. Signs and symptoms of a faint would include:
A) Skin - flushed
B) Pupils - equal, pinpoint
C) Pulse - feeble
D) Breathing - deep, noisy

470. Usually sudden infant death syndrome occurs:
A) Age 1-9 months
B) Age 1-6 months
C) Age 1-10 months
D) Age 1-15 months

471. If an eye injury involves chemicals, should you:
A) Cover the eye with a pad
B) Flush both eyes with copious amounts of water
C) Flush affected eye with copious amounts of water
D) Leave well alone until hospitalisation

472. Neonatal resuscitation should be carried out at a rate of:
A) 120 chest compressions, 40 breaths per minute
B) 80 chest compressions, 20 breaths per minute
C) 80 chest compressions, 40 breaths per minute
D) Any of the above

473. What position would be most comfortable for an appendicitis patient?
A) Prone position
B) Recumbent position
C) Fowler position
D) Trendelenberg position

474. Which of the following is NOT a classification of bones?
A) Long
B) Irregular
C) Flat
D) Sphenoid

475. The kidneys:
A) Produce insulin
B) Regulate salt balance
C) Produce adrenaline
D) Produce bile

476. The length of the oesophagus in a normal adult is:
A) 10-14cm
B) 16-20cm
C) 22-28cm
D) 30-40cm

477. Which of the following is NOT a sign or symptom of pre-eclampsia?
A) Hypotension
B) Protein in the urine
C) Headache
D) Oedema

478. The functions of the liver do NOT include:
A) Detoxifying drugs and poisons
B) Breaking down stored fats
C) Producing adrenaline
D) Producing bile

479. Several organs joined by tracts and vessels are called a system.

480. The lungs are divided by the mediastinum.

481. The right lung contains 3 lobes.

482. The uterus lies between the bladder and the rectum.

483. The humerus joins the scapula at the glenoidal cavity.

484. The uterine arteries are branches of the abdominal aorta.

485. Graafian follicles contain the ova.

486. The second stage of labour is usually hailed by the "breaking of the waters".

487. Physiology is the study of how an organ or system functions.

488. Under normal circumstances the third stage of labour should last no longer than 30 minutes.

489. The respiratory system helps to regulate the acid base balance of the blood.

490. At birth the foramen ovale closes and becomes the fossa ovalis.

491. The placenta will protect the foetus from rubella.

492. Crowning is described as being the birth of the baby's shoulders.

493. The nucleus carries the hereditary factors of the cell called genes.

494. The knee cap or patella is an example of a sesamoid bone.

495. There are 5 different groups of tissues.

496. The oropharynx is shared by both the respiratory and digestive systems.

497. There are two umbilical arteries.

498. The safety of the person attending to the patient must take priority over all else.

499. Infection rarely accompanies a burn.

500. The Glasgow Coma Scale is used to assess the patient's level of consciousness.

501. The mechanism of injury means "how did it happen".

502. You should elevate a wounded limb to reduce blood flow.

503. Foreign objects must be removed from a wound prior to dressing it.

504. The ratio of compressions to inflations when carrying out CPR on a baby is 5-1.

505. The rate of compressions in CPR is 100 per minute.

506. You should be able to palpate a pulse distal to a fracture site.

507. A sign is something the patient can tell you about their condition.

508. The 3 factors used to make a patient assessment are history, signs and observations.

509. Blisters associated with burns must always be burst immediately.

510. The patient's safety comes before your own.

511. The recovery position will help to prevent the inhalation of vomit.

512. The first function to be assessed is breathing in a primary survey.

513. The abdominal cavity houses the lungs.

514. Glands with ducts secrete hormones.

515. A fracture should be immobilised above and below the fracture site.

516. The vertebral column is made up of 32 irregular bones.

517. The cranium is made up of 9 bones.

518. Lateral means towards the midline of the body.

519. The skeletal system comprises 206 bones.

520. A primary survey is carried out to ascertain that life exists and can be sustained.

521. There are 3 types of muscle tissue.

522. A poison can be absorbed into the body.

523. Abnormal pupillary reaction can be indicative of head injury.

524. Plasma is constructed of 90% water and 10% dissolved substances.

525. The patients stomach contents will be extremely alkaline.

526. A symptom is what the patient feels.

527. The nasal cavity warms, moistens and filters incoming air.

528. Nausea is not a sign of shock.

529. The skin has 5 layers.

530. Very little or no precautions need to be taken when transporting a category 1 infectious disease.

531. The control centre that regulates food intake lies within the hypothalamus.

532. Vitamin B3 is derived from meat, liver and flour.

533. Vitamin A is derived from liver, eggs, fish and dairy produce.

534. Vitamin B12 is a fat soluble vitamin.

535. Calcium and iron are essential minerals.

536. Arginine is an essential amino acid.

537. Hypertension may be a predisposing factor of a CVA.

538. Scabies is a category 1 infectious disease.

539. The large intestine is approximately 1.5m long.

540. Approximately 40 people die each year from electrocution.

541. Epilepsy may result from a head injury.

542. Swelling of the throat will cause airway obstruction.

543. The abdominal thrust can be used on infants.

544. The patient in respiratory arrest can still exhibit a pulse.

545. When recording a blood pressure the lower reading is the diastolic.

546. Chickenpox is a category 1 infectious disease.

547. The expression for a full term pregnant woman is primigravida.

548. Airway and C-spine check forms part of a primary survey.

549. When using the Glasgow Coma Scale the best motor response scores 6.

550. Bilateral pupil constriction may be indicative of narcotic overdose.

551. Kinematics of injury deals with obvious injury causes.

552. Hyperglycaemia means low volume of blood sugar.

553. An ectopic pregnancy means the embryo is developing somewhere other than the womb.

554. Difficulty in swallowing is called dysplegia.

555. The placenta is approximately 2.5cm in thickness.

556. The stomach lies within the left lumbar region.

557. A burn is defined as a breach in the continuity of a tissue caused by excessive heat energy.

558. A person less than 20 years of age will usually survive a 20% burn.

559. Using the rule of nines for an adult, one whole leg represents 9% body area.

560. Using the rule of nines for a child, one whole arm represents 18% body area.

561. Normal body temperature is within the range of 36-37°c.

562. Abortion means the expulsion of the foetus before the 14th week of pregnancy.

563. Neurogenic shock occurs as a result of severe haemorrhage.

564. Childbirth consists of 3 stages.

565. Asthma is indicated by an infection of the alveoli.

566. Haem is an iron containing pigment.

567. Plasma is 45% of total blood volume.

568. Anthrax is a category 3 infectious disease.

569. A hypoglycaemic patient is suffering a deficiency of glucose in the blood.

570. Cavitation is associated with pot holing incidents.

571. A patient suffering from a heart attack will always want to lie down.

572. Haemorrhage is a sign of a patient's condition.

573. Hyperglycaemia has a slow onset.

574. A Glasgow Coma Score verbal response of "confused" will record a score of 5.

575. Angina pectoris occurs when coronary circulation is compromised.

576. The spinal cord in an average adult is about 12 inches long.

577. The cerebellum is the largest part of the brain.

578. Parasympathetic dominance has an overall slowing down effect.

579. There are 32 pairs of spinal nerves.

580. Assessment of a patients level of consciousness takes precedence over their ability to breathe.

581. A grand mal seizure is described as having two stages.

582. Stroke volume in the average adult is 95ml.

583. The wall of the heart is made up of two layers of tissue.

584. Oxygen and carbon dioxide are exchanged within the alveoli of the lungs.

585. The mitral or bicuspid valve is situated between the left atria and the left ventricle.

586. The left ventricle of the heart pumps blood to the lungs.

587. The normal respiratory rate for an adult is 16-20 times per minute.

588. A fractured pelvis will usually result in incontinence.

589. The brachial pulse is used to assess the heartbeat of small children and infants.

590. Cardiac output = Stroke volume x Heart rate.

591. The Glasgow Coma Score for “extensor response” is 3.

592. Pulmonary circulation removes blood from the liver.

593. Tunica media is the elastic muscular layer of a blood vessel.

594. Thrombocytes fight infection.

595. Erythrocytes number approximately 9,000 per cubic millimetre of blood.

596. Nausea is a symptom of a patient’s condition.

597. A Glasgow Coma response of “eyes open to pain” will record a score of 2.

598. Direct pressure should not be applied to an open wound containing a foreign object.

599. A contused wound is caused by a sharp knife.

600. The area of the brain which registers crude sensations of pain is the thalamus.

601. A hypoglycaemic patient may appear uncoordinated, confused, aggressive and drunk.

602. The pleura is made up of three layers.

603. Both lungs have three lobes.

604. Patients with chronic bronchitis should always be given high concentrations of oxygen therapy.

605. Neurones can either be afferent or efferent.

606. One of the functions of CSF is to supply food to certain cells of the brain.

607. The dura mater is the tough outermost layer that covers the brain and spinal cord.

608. The pia mater is a delicate membrane which closely covers the brain.

609. Hypoxaemia means low oxygen content in arterial blood.

610. A patient suffering a head injury and showing signs of shock must have other injuries.

611. The first line in paraquat poisoning is to administer oxygen.

612. Whooping cough is a category II infectious disease.

613. Entonox is composed of 50% oxygen and 50% nitrous oxide.

614. The spinal cord receives and relays impulses to and from the cranial nerves.

615. 1 in 20 children will be born with some abnormality or defect.

616. A normal persons centre of gravity is anterior to the base of the spine.

617. Patients with chest injuries should be positioned semi-recumbent, inclined to the injured side.

618. If it is difficult to maintain an unconscious patient's airway, you should raise the legs and lower the head.

619. Patients with spinal injuries should always be transported in the supine position with a pillow supporting the head.

620. Head injured patients should always be placed in the recumbent position.

621. There are 8 carpal bones in the wrist.

622. There are 14 phalanges in the foot.

623. Ligaments are non-elastic fibres attaching muscles to bones.

624. A strain is a tearing or wrenching of a ligament.

625. Chemicals are produced in three physical forms.

626. Entonox can be given to a patient with a closed pneumothorax.

627. Patients suffering carbon monoxide poisoning require very little oxygen.

628. Phenobarbitone is taken to control epilepsy.

629. A patient in status epilepticus should not be given oxygen.

630. The lowest Glasgow Coma Score is 0.

631. In a contre-coup injury, the injury to the brain is on the same side as the external skull injury.

632. Compression can be caused by intercranial haemorrhage.

633. One dilated pupil and one normal pupil will indicate injury on the dilated side.

634. Burns in excess of 10% are considered to be serious.

635. The normal body core temperature is approximately 39°C.

636. Rabies is a category 1 infectious disease.

637. A burn covering both the patient's head and neck constitutes 9% of the body surface area.

638. The endometrium is the outer layer of the uterus.

639. Not all fractures require formal splintage.

640. The respiratory centre is situated in the cerebrum.

641. The left bronchus is narrower than the right.

642. Vessels enter and leave the lung at the hilum.

643. Hypoxia is a result of too much oxygen.

644. Nerve impulses from the respiratory centre pass via the phrenic nerve to the diaphragm.

645. The respiratory centre of a chronic bronchitic is stimulated by raised carbon dioxide levels in the blood.

646. A chronic asthmatic will have difficulty expiring.

647. Haemothorax is air in the pleural cavity.

648. Eclampsia is potentially life threatening for both baby and mother.

649. The middle layer of the heart wall is called the myocardium.

650. The right atrium and ventricle are divided by the tricuspid valve.

651. The best possible Glasgow Coma Score is 10.

652. Multipolar neurones are usually afferent.

653. Approximately 500 people die from burns each year.

654. With regard to the rule of nines, one adult arm is equal to 18% of the body area.

655. The patient's hand is equal to 1% of the body area.

656. The epidermis is responsible for skin colour and waterproofing.

657. Partial thickness burns are divided into three categories.

658. Hyperglycaemia has a sudden onset.

659. Infectious diseases can be spread through indirect contact.

660. Excessive bleeding after the birth of a baby is called postpartum haemorrhage.

661. Vomiting must be induced in all types of poisoning.

662. Bipolar neurones are usually sensory in function.

663. There are four types of fracture.

664. Approximately 1 in 200 people have some form of mental illness.

665. There are two main types of mental illness.

666 Neurotransmitters are responsible for passing on impulses from one neurone to another.

667. When lifting, your head should be raised, looking forward.

668. The cerebrum is divided into three hemispheres.

669. A cerebral hemisphere is divided into four lobes.

670. Head injured patients should be placed in the recumbent position.

671. The patella is the largest sesamoid bone.

672. All bones are covered in peritoneum.

673. There are 16 facial bones and 8 cranial bones making up the skull.

674. The zygoma and zygomatic arch are found in the ear.

675. There are 8 tarsal bones in the ankle.

676. There are 18 phalanges in the hand.

677. Disabled people can be registered disabled by the Department of Employment.

678. Inspired air contains 16% oxygen.

679. AIDS stands for Acquired Immune Deficiency System.

680. A symptom of a fractured pelvis is the urge to pass urine.

681. If you are not sure that a fracture is present it is best to leave it alone.

682. Blood consists of 55% plasma and 45% solids.

683. Angina pectoris may develop into myocardial infarction.

684. Blood cells involved with fighting infection are called platelets.

685. Arteries carry blood away from the heart.

686. Veins and arteries are made up of three layers.

687. The adult heart weighs approximately 8-11 ounces.

688. Venous blood is bright red in colour and will spurt from a wound.

689. A hypovolaemic patient will display a slow, full pulse.

690. The skin is responsible for the reception of stimuli.

691. A radial pulse can be located at the wrist.

692. The skin provides a protective barrier against infection.

693. The nervous system consists mainly of the brain and spinal cord.

694. Each neurone has three component parts.

695. The membranes that surround the brain are called the pleura.

696. The brain can be divided into four main parts.

697. A fitting epileptic patient should always be restrained.

698. The spinal cord is approximately 12-18 inches long.

699. There are 42 pairs of spinal nerves.

700. The peripheral nervous system is divided into two sections.

701. The patient with a spinal injury must always be placed in the recovery position.

702. A petit mal only lasts a few seconds.

703. An indication of a fracture is the sound made when testing for crepitus.

704. A tourniquet should be applied to arrest haemorrhage.

705. Bone is surrounded by periosteum.

706. A grand mal seizure has only four stages.

707. Axons transmit impulses away from the cell body.

708. The diencephalon consists of the thalamus and the hypothalamus.

709. The parasympathetic system is responsible for creating the conditions associated with sleep.

710. Periosteum is a dense white fibrous covering around the surface of the bone.

711. The transformation of embryonic tissues into bone is called ossification.

712. Bone is 30-40% water.

713. Red bone marrow is responsible for producing blood cells.

714. The femur is classified as a flat bone.

715. A petit mal has four stages.

716. Oxygen enters the blood by diffusion.

717. The respiratory rate of a healthy infant is 32-40 breaths per minute.

718. Internal respiration takes place in the lungs.

719. The medulla oblongata is concerned with the voluntary movement of muscles.

720. Haversian canals are found in bones.

721. Asthma may result from an allergy.

722. The skin is involved with the control of body temperature.

723. A gliding joint allows freedom of movement in all directions.

724. The inflation to compression ratio in two man CPR is 5-1.

725. Oropharyngeal airways will protect the lungs from inhalation of vomit.

726. An asphyxiated patient must NOT be given high levels of oxygen.

727. External respiration takes place in the tissues.

728. Expired air contains 16% oxygen.

729. A lobule is the smallest anatomical portion of the lung.

730. The outermost layer of the meninges is the dura mater.

731. A greenstick fracture usually occurs in the elderly.

732. The epiglottis lies in the nasal cavity.

733. As air is taken into the body it is dried.

734. As we breathe in the diaphragm contracts.

735. The respiratory centre lies in the chest.

736. The patient in cardiac arrest will have a weak pulse.

737. In adult CPR the ratio of inflations to compressions for one operator is 2 to 15.

738. Bronchial asthma is a non reversible condition.

739. Chemoreceptors measure the amount of carbon monoxide in the blood.

740. Hypoxic drive is the stimulation to breathe by low oxygen levels in the blood.

741. The periosteum has no blood supply.

742. Tidal volume in the average adult is 600ml.

743. The face is made up of eight bones.

744. Once a fracture has been reduced by applying traction, traction should be reduced to prevent further pain at the injury site.

745. Immobilising a fracture will help prevent further damage.

746. A dislocation can look similar to a fracture.

747. You only need to check the pulse proximal to the injury.

748. A simple or closed fracture will have an external wound.

749. Cords of fibrous tissue which attach muscles to bones are called tendons.

750. A ball and socket joint allows for flexion and extension in one direction only.

751. The larynx is also shared by the digestive tract.

752. The left lung has 3 lobes.

753. The trachea has 16-20 C-shaped rings of cartilage along its length.

754. The pleura is a serous membrane.

755. The epiglottis is a leaf shaped flap of cartilage.

756. Short bones develop from cartilage tissue.

757. A left sided heart failure is usually secondary to right sided failure.

758. A burn of 10% of the body area may produce signs and symptoms of shock.

759. An unconscious CVA patient should be nursed in the recovery position, paralysed side down.

760. A faint is often referred to as apoplexy.

761. Haemodialysis patients may become hypertensive.

762. In normal labour the second stage takes the longest.

763. When dealing with a suspected child abuse case you should let the parent know that you do not believe their account of the incident.

764. In a premature baby the skull may appear unduly small.

765. If during labour there is a prolapsed cord the patient should be transported face down in the Trendelenberg position.

766. A CVA may be caused by a blocked cerebral blood vessel.

767. Superficial burns can cause redness and blistering causing nerve damage.

768. Entonox cylinders are blue with a white neck.

769. A patient's hand is equal to 5% of body area.

770. Patients with heart conditions are a high risk group for suffering shock.

771. Ischaemic heart failure is an acute condition.

772. Patients with congestive cardiac failure should always be transported recum bent to aid blood flow.

773. An insect sting could lead to severe shock.

774. A spinal injury could lead to severe shock.

775. A thin film of serous fluid separates the dura and arachnoid mater.

776. The length of the spinal cord in the average adult is approximately 24 inches.

777. Axons transmit impulses towards the cell body.

778. Within the brain, cell bodies are known as grey matter.

779. Reflex centres involved in swallowing and vomiting lie within the thalamus.

780. CSF is produced in the choroid plexuses within the ventricles of the brain.

781. The autonomic nervous system controls involuntary muscle contraction.

782. Boiling water and fat tend to cool quickly and cause less skin damage.

783. The small intestine is approximately 8-9 metres in length.

784. The pharynx is divided into three parts.

785. A yankeur catheter can be inserted into the pharynx.

786. Flexible catheters should be stored folded.

787. The inflation rate for small babies in respiratory arrest is 32-40 per minute.

788. Asphyxia can be caused by poisoning.

789. Premature neonates require copious amounts of oxygen.

790. Internal respiration takes place in the lungs.

791. Entonox is an analgesic gas formed of oxygen and carbon dioxide.

792. If there is too much carbon dioxide in the blood the pH will fall.

793. Dyspnoea means difficulty in breathing.

794. A motor cyclist's helmet should be removed by only one member of the crew.

795. Angina is an acute condition.

796. The cardiac sphincter can be found in the stomach.

797. A patient suffering from shock may respond better if given a drink of warm tea.

798. A patient will become diabetic after having their pancreas removed.

799. A respiratory rate of less then 10 or more than 29 is an indication for IPPV.

800. Anaerobic means with oxygen.

801. Chest pain is not always a symptom of myocardial infarction.

802. Parkinson's disease is a brain malfunction that deals with involuntary muscle movement.

803. There are 4 pulmonary veins carrying blood to the lungs.

804. Fibrin is a plasma protein.

805. A lacerated wound is usually made by a sharp edged object.

806. Blood volume is 70 ml per kg body weight.

807. To guarantee a patent airway in an unconscious patient an oropharyngeal airway must be inserted.

808. A strain is a tearing or wrenching of a ligament.

809. To aid digestion, the stomach contains hydrochloric acid.

810. What **A** is a gradual loss of elasticity of the artery walls?

811. What **A** is a local dilation of a blood vessel?

812. What **A** is a loss of memory?

813. What **A** is a piece of suction apparatus?

814. What **A** is a type of drug used to treat mental illness?

815. What **A** is the absence of oxygen within the body tissue?

816. What **A** is the cessation of breathing?

817. What **A** is the location of a Potts fracture?

818. What **A** is the medical term for armpit?

819. What **A** is the technique of listening and interpreting sounds that occur in the body with a stethoscope?

820. What **B** aids the breakdown of chyme?

821. What **B** is a delivery where the baby's bottom emerges before the head?

822. What **B** is a haemorrhage that may occur during a cerebrovascular accident?

823. What **B** is a popular name for decompression sickness?

824. What **B** is a term that means affecting both sides of the body?

825. What **B** is a valve that connects left atrium and left ventricle of the heart?

826. What **B** is an abnormally slow heart rate below 60 bpm?

827. What **B** is inflammation of the bronchi?

828. What **B** is the artery used to record a pulse in babies?

829. What **B** rises into the hypogastric region when full?

830. What **C** are selectively opened and closed depending on the body's demand for blood flow?

831. What **C** is a clear watery fluid that circulates between the ventricles within the brain, the meninges and the central canal in the spinal cord?

832. What **C** is a developing sign of patients suffering from increasing hypoxia?

833. What **C** is a fracture associated with the wrist?

834. What **C** is a pulse that should be felt for in a collapsed patient?

835. What **C** is a region of the brain concerned primarily with the maintenance of posture and balance and with the coordination of movement?

836. What **C** is a term that means pertaining to the heart and blood vessels?

837. What **C** is an accident often termed a stroke?

838. What **C** is an output that can be increased by up to twelve times during exercise?

839. What **C** is the first and widest part of the large intestine?

840. What **D** is a condition in which a person's water content has fallen to a dangerously low level?

841. What **D** is a disorder caused by insufficient or absent production of the hormone insulin by the pancreas?

842. What **D** is a side effect of Entonox?

843. What **D** is a symptom of neuroses and psychoses?

844. What **D** is a term describing a part of the body that is further away from an other part?

845. What **D** is difficult or laboured breathing?

846. What **D** is the largest muscle of respiration?

847. What **D** is the medical term for profuse sweating?

848. What **D** is the period when the heart is at rest?

849. What **E** is a blockage of an artery by a fragment of material travelling in the bloodstream?

850. What **E** is a disease in which the alveoli in the lungs become damaged?

851. What **E** is a form of pregnancy or an abnormal heart contraction?

852. What **E** is a medical term for nosebleed?

853. What **E** is a rare but serious condition of late pregnancy characterised by convulsions and sometimes coma or death?

854. What **E** is any condition that requires immediate medical treatment?

855. What **E** is the escape of fluid through the walls of a blood vessel into a tissue or body cavity?

856. What **E** is the inner lining of the heart?

857. What **E** is the unborn child during the first eight weeks of pregnancy?

858. What **F** is another word for tiredness?

859. What **F** is described as chaotic electrical activity within the myocardium?

860. What **F** is that of the phonetic alphabet?

861. What **F** is the common term for syncope?

862. What **F** is the convulsing common to young children?

863. What **F** is the main artery of the leg?

864. What **F** is the medical term for the thigh bone?

865. What **F** is the seventh cranial nerve?

866. What **F** is the stretcher position recommended for abdominal pain?

867. What **F** is the tube that extends from the uterus to the ovary?

868. What **F** is the unborn child from the end of the eighth week after conception to birth?

869. What **F** is the waste material from the digestive tract?

870. What **G** is a branch of medicine concerned with the elderly?

871. What **G** is a condition in which the pressure of fluid in the eye is so high that it causes damage?

872. What **G** is a group of specialised cells that manufacture and release chemical substances such as hormones and enzymes?

873. What **G** is a unit of the material of heredity?

874. What **G** is the drug administered to hypoglycaemic patients?

875. What **G** is the inflammation of the stomach and intestines?

876. What **G** is the ninth cranial nerve?

877. What **G** is the period from conception to birth during which the developing infant is carried in the uterus?

878. What **G** is the small pear shaped sac situated underneath the liver?

879. What **G** is the soft tissue condition that may occur due to lack of oxygen and infection?

880. What **H** is a localised collection of blood caused by bleeding from ruptured capillaries?

881. What **H** is an inherited bleeding disorder caused by a deficiency of a particular blood protein?

882. What **H** is the bone of the upper arm?

883. What **H** is the destruction of red blood cells?

884. What **H** is the medical term for bleeding?

885. What **H** is the medical term for coughing up blood?

886. What **H** is the medical term for vomiting blood?

887. What **H** is the oxygen carrying pigment found in red blood cells?

888. What **H** is the presence of blood in the urine?

889. What **H** is the removal of waste products from the blood by means of artificial filtration?

890. What **H** is the shock that may be present in a patient who has lost a large amount of body fluid?

891. What **H** is the study of blood and its formation?

892. What **I** is a hormone produced by the pancreas?

893. What **I** is a term usually applied to a baby up to the age of 12 months?

894. What **I** is redness, swelling, heat and pain in a tissue due to injury or infection?

895. What **I** is the apparatus in which premature infants are placed in and used to transport them between hospitals?

896. What **I** is the death of an area of cardiac tissue caused by a lack of blood supply?

897. What **I** is the final, longest and narrowest section of the small intestine?

898. What **I** is the inability to produce offspring?

899. What **I** is the system of the body concerned with fighting infection?

900. What **I** is the technique used to prevent movement of joints of bones?

901. What **I** is the uncontrollable, involuntary passing of urine?

902. What **J** describes the edge of a lacerated wound?

903. What **J** is a disorder of the liver characterised by yellowing of the skin and whites of the eyes?

904. What **J** is one of three veins on each side of the neck that return deoxygenated blood from the head to the heart?

905. What **J** is the international unit of energy, work and heat?

906. What **J** is the junction between two or more bones?

907. What **J** is the middle, coiled section of the small intestine joining the duodenum to the ileum?

908. What **J** is the only moveable bone in the face?

909. What **K** is a potentially serious condition characterised by sweet, fruity smelling breath and associated with hyperglycaemia?

910. What **K** is an organ to which the adrenal gland is attached?

911. What **K** is the common name for the patella?

912. What **K** is the medical term for excessive backward curvature of the spine?

913 What **K** is the name given to breathing in ketoacidosis characterised by hyperpnoea and tachypnoea?

914 What **K** is the study of movement, important in lifting and transferring?

915 What **L** is a method of directly examining the interior of the abdomen by means of a viewing instrument?

916 What **L** is a torn, irregular wound?

917 What **L** is a tough fibrous band of tissue which binds joints together?

918 What **L** is a weak acid produced when cells breakdown glucose by anaerobic metabolism to produce energy?

919 What **L** is any type of white blood cell?

920 What **L** is the common name for the lower limbs?

921 What **L** is the medical term for the voice box?

922 What **L** is the term for inflammation of the larynx?

923 What **L** means relating to or situated on, one side?

924 What **M** are the three membranes that cover and protect the brain and spinal cord?

925 What **M** is a cell which is present in most body tissues, that plays an important role in allergies?

926 What **M** is a medical term meaning towards the midline of the body?

927 What **M** is black, tarry faeces caused by internal bleeding?

928 What **M** is one of a pair of bones that forms the upper jaw?

929 What **M** is the medical term for paralysis of one limb?

930 What **M** is the medical term for the lower jaw?

931 What **M** is the middle layer of the heart?

932 What **M** is the process of chewing food?

933 What **M** is the space between the lungs?

934. What **N** is a device used to administer Salbutamol?

935. What **N** is a form of shock which affects the control of blood vessels?

936. What **N** is a newly born infant under the age of one month?

937. What **N** is a state of stupor, which is usually caused by a drug?

938. What **N** is inflammation of the kidneys?

939. What **N** is the death of tissue cells?

940. What **N** is the location of the carotid pulse?

941. What **N** is the microscopic unit of the kidneys?

942. What **N** is the passage connecting the nasal cavity behind the nose to the top of the throat behind the soft palate?

943. What **N** is the sensation of needing to vomit?

944. What **N** is the system of the body concerned with information?

945. What **O** is a branch of medicine concerned with child birth?

946. What **O** is a substance obtained from the unripe seed pods of the poppy plant?

947. What **O** is an abnormal accumulation of fluid in the body tissues?

948. What **O** is the branch of surgery concerned with disorders of the bones and joints and their associated muscles, tendons and ligaments?

949. What **O** is the first cranial nerve?

950. What **O** is the muscular tube that carries food from the throat to the stomach?

951. What **O** is the passage of a solvent (e.g. water) through a semipermeable membrane from a weaker solution to a stronger solution?

952. What **O** is the third cranial nerve?

953. What **P** is a medical term applied to a disease that occurs over a large geographical area and affects a high proportion of the population?

954. What **P** is a poisonous weedkiller?

955. What **P** is a sensation that can range from mild discomfort to an unbearable and excruciating experience?

956. What **P** is an abnormal paleness of the skin and mucous membranes, particularly discernible in the face?

957. What **P** is an awareness of one's heartbeat or a sensation of having a rapid and unusually forceful beat?

958. What **P** is an external device that supplies electrical impulses to the heart to maintain the heartbeat at a regular rate?

959. What **P** is the branch of medicine concerned with the growth and development of children?

960. What **P** is the nervous system that controls the involuntary activities of the organs, glands, blood vessels and other tissues in the body?

961. What **P** is the paralysis of both legs?

962. What **P** is where the islets of Langerhans are found?

963. What **R** describes the return of swallowed food or drink into the oesophagus or mouth?

964. What **R** is a viral infection also known as German measles?

965. What **R** is joined to the sternum and vertebrae?

966. What **R** is sometimes detached in trauma to the eye?

967. What **R** is the emission of energy in the form of waves or particles?

968. What **R** is the medical term meaning related to the kidneys?

969. What **R** is the pain felt in a part of the body at some distance from its cause?

970. What **R** is the position used for an unconscious patient?

971. What **R** is the recurrence of a disease after an apparent recovery?

972. What **S** is a bronchodilator drug used in the treatment of asthma?

973. What **S** is a burn caused by hot liquid or steam?

974. What **S** is a dangerous reduction of blood from throughout the body tissues which if untreated, may lead to collapse, coma or even death?

975. What **S** is a dividing wall that separates the left and right chambers of the heart?

976. What **S** is a tearing or stretching of the ligaments?

977. What **S** is the anatomical name for the shoulder blade?

978. What **S** is the most common form of psychosis?

979. What **S** is the nerve to avoid when administering Glucagon via the buttocks?

980. What **S** is the organ that removes and destroys worn out red blood cells?

981. What **S** is the period when the heart is contracting?

982. What **T** is a blood clot that has formed inside an intact blood vessel?

983. What **T** is a disease often referred to by the letters TB?

984. What **T** is a drug used in short term treatment of insomnia and often taken as an overdose?

985. What **T** is a heart rate above 100 beats per minute?

986. What **T** is an abnormally fast rate of breathing?

987. What **T** is an artery that runs anterior to the ear?

988. What **T** is another name for quadriplegia?

989. What **T** is likely to deviate in a patient presenting with a tension pneumothorax?

990. What **T** is the compression of the heart due to a collection of fluid under the lining?

991. What **T** is the inner and thicker of the two long bones in the lower leg?

992. What **T** is the medical name for the chest?

993. What **U** is a skin condition, also known as nettle rash or hives, characterised by the development of raised white or yellow lumps surrounded by an area of red inflammation?

994. What **U** is a system of the body that deals with the disposal of waste products?

995. What **U** is one of the bones of the forearm?

996. What **U** is the cord connecting the foetus to the placenta that supplies oxygen and nutrients from the mother's circulation?

997. What **U** is the tube by which urine is passed from the bladder?

998. What **W** is a common injury in RTA's which should be treated as serious until proven otherwise?

999. What **W** is a high pitched, whistling sound produced in the chest during breathing which is caused by narrowing of the airways?

1000. What **W** is an anticoagulant drug used to treat and prevent abnormal blood clotting?

Answers

1 A
2 A
3 C
4 D
5 D
6 B

A respiratory assessment consists of inspection, palpation, auscultation and persussion.

7 D
8 C

Inspection, palpation and percussion are physical assessment techniques, pallor is a sign.

9 A
10 D
11 A
12 D
13 C
14 A
15 B
16 D
17 C
18 B
19 A
20 A
21 C
22 A
23 B
24 C
25 D

Remember the gauge is inversely proportional to the diameter.

26 B
27 A
28 D
29 C
30 D
31 A
32 B
33 D

Thrombocytes are involved in the clotting process, the others are leukocytes involved in fighting infection.

34 C
35 D
36 B
37 B
38 D

The others are types of nerve - sensory (afferent), motor (efferent).

39 B
40 B
41 D

Pia mater is the inner layer of the meninges, the others are parts of the brain.

42 A
43 C
44 A
45 A
46 A
47 C
48 C
49 B
50 B
51 A

The other three are part of the coronary circulation.

52 B
53 B
54 C
55 D

A haemothorax patient should be transported injured side down to minimise complication of the injury.

56 D

Dextrose 50% is a hypertonic solution.

57 A
58 D
59 C

Aspirin would be part of the treatment for an MI but oxygen would be more appropriate in the initial stages of assessment.

60 D
61 A
62 C
63 A
64 A

Distended neck veins is the only relevant sign, choking is a symptom and bradycardia is not associated with circulatory overload.

65 B
66 B

Gelofusine is a colloid.

67 D
68 C

Obviously every intubation is going to be different but as a rule of thumb, if you need to breath so does the patient.

69 C
70 A
71 C
72 B

Pain at the site of an infusion would probably indicate a missed cannulation. The fluid would be infiltrating the local tissues causing pain.

73 C
74 D

Inspiratory reserve is the volume of forced inspiration, vital capacity is the volume taken in by forced inhalation after forced exhalation.

75 D
76 C
77 D
78 True
79 True
80 True
81 False

Patients should only be intubated when it is necessary to protect the airway.

82 False
83 False

Glucagon is secreted by the pancreas.

84 False
The pneumotaxic area is located within the pons varolii.

85 False
86 False
Dead air space comprises all the parts of the respiratory tract through which no diffusion takes place and is filled by 150ml of air.

87 False
Morphine is a respiratory depressant.

88 False
As the air passages divide they contain less cartilage and more smooth muscle.

89 True
90 False
Tachycardia is a sign of LVF.

91 True
92 False
CSF is produced in the ventricles of the brain and reabsorbed in the superior sagittal sinus.

93 True
94 False
The apneustic area is located in the lower pons.

95 False
The liver secretes prothrombin.

96 False
The stroke volume is the amount of blood pumped at each contraction.

97 False
The cardioacceleratory centre is stimulated by noradrenaline, the cardioinhibitory centre is stimulated by acetylcholine.

98 True
99 True
100 True

101 False
Leukocytes increase in number during times of infection.

102 True
The two divisions of the peripheral nervous system are the sympathetic and parasympathetic.

103 False
The cardiac cycle takes 0.8 seconds.

104 False
The medulla oblongata is 2.5cm long and is shaped like a pyramid with its base upper-most.

105 True
106 False
Hypovolaemia means low volume of blood which is an indication for fluid replacement.

107 True
108 True
109 False
Sodium bicarbonate can only be administered via a patent IV cannula.

110 True
111 True
112 True
113 False
The SA node is situated high in the right atria.

114 False
Antepartum means before birth, postpartum is after birth.

115 False
116 False
Stroke volume is the amount of blood ejected from either ventricle at each contraction. Cardiac output is the amount of blood ejected from either ventricle per minute.

117 False
The 3 lead ECG is based on Einthoven's triangle.

118 False
The normal firing rate of the SA node is 60-80 beats per minute.

119 False
The aVR lead is placed on the right arm.

120 True
121 True
122 False
Bradycardia indicates a rate below 60 beats per minute.

123 True
124 True
125 False
There are 4 grades of difficulty to patient intubation based on anatomical shape and visible glottis area.

126 True
127 True
Strictly speaking the alveoli become infected and inflamed hampering gaseous diffusion across the alveolar-capillary membrane.

128 True
129 True
130 True
131 False
There are terminal bronchioles and alveolar ducts between the bronchioles and alveoli.

132 False
Horizontal lines on ECG paper represent amplitude, vertical lines represent time.

133 True
134 True
135 True
136 True

137 False
Shock can be severe in an ectopic pregnancy due to concealed haemorrhage.

138 False
Adrenaline is a naturally occurring substance.

139 False
Atropine is a parasympathetic blocking agent.

140 True
141 False
142 True
143 False
The cardiac output is increased by 20-30% in the second trimester of pregnancy.

144 False
145 True
146 False
Hartmann's is a crystalloid solution.

147 True
148 False
Pregnant women are more prone to vaso-vagal attacks due to the physiological changes to the respiratory and cardiovascular systems during pregnancy.

149 True
150 False
Sodium bicarbonate is an alkaline solution.

151 False
Chest palpation is carried out with the hands, a stethoscope can be used for chest auscultation.

152 True
153 True
154 True

155 False
The orifice is called the foramen ovale.

156 True
157 True
158 True
159 False
Short muscular necks constitute one of the major anatomical difficulties of intubation.

160 False
161 C
162 C
163 C
164 B
MFIs are very prone to airway obstruction because of unstable bones, blood loss, broken teeth, numbness.

165 A
Oxygen yokes have two pins.

166 C
167 A
Entonox will leak into the interpleural space easier than other gases so must not be used in severe chest injury e.g. pneumothorax.

168 B
169 C
170 B
Skeletal, smooth and cardiac.

171 B
172 D
173 C
A flow meter regulates the flow of oxygen to the patient. A humidifier is used to moisten the oxygen supplied to a patient.

174 D
The maxilla is regarded as an irregular bone, whereas the others are long bones.

175 C
176 A
The stomach, duodenum, kidneys and large intestines all lie within the abdominal cavity.

177 B
The pharynx is divided into the nasopharynx, oropharynx and laryngopharynx.

178 C
The cricoid is a cartilage within the larynx, the carina is at the very base of the trachea and the mediastinum is a tissue mass that separates the lungs.

179 C
The pH scale measures from 0 (highly acidic) to 14 (highly alkaline). 7 is neutral, neither acidic nor alkaline, therefore blood at 7.4 is slightly alkaline.

180 B
Inspired oxygen comprises 20% of air. Inspired carbon dioxide comprises 0.04% on inspiration and 4% on expiration.

181 A
Tachypnoea is an increased respiratory rate, cyanosis is a blue disolouration seen in hypoxia which is a lack of oxygen to the tissues.

182 B
Because the pressure in the cranial vault is gradually increasing the signs and symptoms take time to build up. The other answers are classic signs of hypovolaemic shock.

183 A
184 A
185 A
Spaces within the cranium are called sinuses.

186 A
Looking from the outer layer to the inner, the sequence is dura, arachnoid then pia.

187 A
188 C
189 C
The spinal nerves consist of 8 pairs cervical, 12 pairs thoracic, 5 pairs lumbar, 5 pairs sacral, 1 pair coccygeal.

190 A
191 C
Clotting factors are found in blood and not cerebrospinal fluid.

192 C
193 C
Airway, Breathing, Circulation, Disability.

194 D
195 C
196 A
197 D
The femur is in the leg, the others are in the arm.

198 B
199 D
200 C
The eyes move together so if you leave the good eye open the bad eye will move when the patient looks around. If you cover both eyes the patient should keep them still.

201 C
202 C
NEVER apply creams to a burn. They only have to be painfully removed in Casualty.

203 D
204 B
205 B
206 D
In the rule of nines for an adult the front and back of the torso are both equal to 18%.

207 B
208 B
Asthma is associated with a difficulty in EXHALING along with coughing and dyspnoea. Inspiratory wheezing is generally caused by upper airway obstructions.

209 A
210 A
211 A
212 C
The meninges have 3 layers, the dura mater (outer layer), arachnoid mater (middle) and pia mater (inner).

213 B
214 A
The diaphysis is the shaft and the periosteum is a fibrous vascular covering.

215 D
7 true ribs (connected anteriorly to the sternum), 3 false ribs (connected anteriorly to the rib above) and 2 floating ribs (unattached to anything anterior).

216 B
217 C
Pathological fractures are caused by old age taking its toll on the bones or disease.

218 D
219 A
220 B
221 A

222 C
The others are facial bones, sphenoidal is a cranial bone.

223 D
The tibia is a long bone of the leg, the others are all found in the arm.

224 D
225 B
226 C
227 A
A slow full pulse is a sign of compression.

228 C
Acetone breath is a classic sign of hyperglycaemia.

229 C
Pericardium is the outer layer, myocardium the muscley inner layer. Epicardium is a component of the pericardium.

230 B
231 C
232 A
Hyphema is blood in the eye, haematuria is blood in the urine and haemorrhage is general bleeding.

233 C
234 B
235 B
236 A
237 C
238 B
239 C
240 D
241 B
242 A
243 C
244 B
245 A
246 C
247 D

248 A
249 C
250 D
The pulmonary artery carries deoxygenated blood to the lungs for oxygenation, the others carry oxygenated blood.

251 C
252 C
253 D
254 B
255 C
256 B
257 D
258 A
259 B
260 D
The others are regions of the abdominal cavity.

261 C
The others are part of the cell structure.

262 A
263 C
264 D
265 A
266 A
267 A
268 A
269 D
270 B
271 A
272 B
273 A
274 A
275 D
276 D
277 D
278 C
The oesophagus is associated with digestion, the others with respiration.

279 C
280 A
281 B
282 D
283 B
284 D
285 A
286 D
The mandible is part of the face, the others part of the cranium.

287 A
288 B
289 A
290 B
291 A
292 A
293 A
294 B
295 B
296 C
297 B
298 B
The Fowler is a stretcher position.

299 D
300 B
301 C
The left lung has 2 lobes to accommodate the position of the heart.

302 A
303 C
304 B
305 A
306 C
307 C
308 C
309 B
310 B
311 C
While the organs of respiration are located in the thoracic cavity, the RESPIRATORY CENTRE is located in the medulla oblongata and therefore the cranial cavity.

312 A
313 D
314 C
Pupils dilate when the brain is starved of oxygen.

315 D
Whooping cough is a category I infectious disease, the others are all category III.

316 B
Jaundice is an increase in bile pigmentation taken up by the tissues.

317 D
318 C
319 D
320 D
321 D
322 B
323 C
324 C
325 C
Gene mal does not exist, the others are all types of seizure.

326 D
327 D
328 C
329 A
330 A
331 A
332 B
While it could be argued that in a continuing cycle both A and D could be deemed to be correct, only B is in the correct order.

333 B
334 D
335 C
336 B
337 A
338 C
339 A
340 A
Obeys commands is part of the Glasgow Coma Scale's motor response, the others are from the eye response.

341 C
Skin colour is a sign, the others are symptoms.

342 C
Nausea is a symptom, the others are signs.

343 A
344 A
345 C
346 B
Lumbar is a region not a cavity.

347 C
348 A
349 D
350 B
Blood pressure is reduced in shock.

351 B
352 C
Response related to the eyes is a separate category within the Glasgow Coma Scale.

353 A
Thick yellow-green sputum is associated with infections such as bronchitis.

354 B
355 B
356 A
357 D
The knee cap is a sesamoid bone, all the others are long bones.

358 D
359 D
You can make a diagnosis after you have found information about the others.

360 A
Symptoms are things the patient feels and can tell you about.

361 B
362 C
363 C
364 D
365 B
366 D
367 D
368 C
369 C
370 D
GCS: 1-4 eye, 1-5 verbal, 1-6 motor.

371 A
372 C
373 B
The larynx is the only one in the list which is part of the respiratory system not the digestive system.

374 C
375 B
376 C
377 B
378 A
379 C
380 B
381 A
382 B
383 C
384 B
The axis bone is the 1st cervical vertebrae.

385 C
386 D
387 C
388 D
389 D
390 B
Abdominal is not a pulse point, the others are.

391 C
392 B
393 A
394 B
The air is warmed, not cooled by the nasal cavity.

395 D
396 B
397 D
Never induce vomiting in any poisoning. With Paraquat poisoning it should be encouraged.

398 B
399 A
Fruity breath smell is a sign of hyperglycaemia.

400 D
401 A
402 C
Nothing should be administered orally to a potentially shocked patient.

403 C
404 C
405 B
The others are acidic, quick lime is an alkali.

406 D
407 A
408 D
409 D
The others are conductors or stimulators of impulses, the interventricular septum is an insulator.

410 A
411 C
412 A
413 D
414 D
415 C
Angina pectoris is chest pain when there is inadequate oxygenation of the heart due to a narrowing of the arteries as opposed to a complete blockage in myocardial infarction.

416 A
417 B
418 B
419 A
420 B
421 D
The left ventricle has the thickest layer myocardium because it has work the hardest and has to withstand the most pressure.

422 D
423 D
424 C
425 D
426 B
A slow, full pulse is associated with a head injury.

427 A
428 B
429 B
Infantile convulsions usually occur when the child is too warm.

430 C
431 D
432 C
433 B
The axon carries the impulse away from the cell body.

434 C
435 D
Chickenpox is a category 2 infectious disease.

436 D
Sporadic - scattered or isolated. Epidemic - rapid spread. Pandemic - epidemic which spreads all over the world.

437 B
2.5kg = 5lb.

438 B
439 B
Pupils will dilate due to loss of nervous control.

440 B
Rapid, shallow pulse is a sign of shock.

441 B
442 C
Blood volume is made up of 55% fluid and 45% solids.

443 D
Synovial membranes are associated with joints and synaptic membranes with neurones.

444 B
Since the eyes move in unison you should cover them both to prevent the casualty inadvertently moving the bad eye while looking around.

445 B
446 C
447 B
448 B
The hypothalamus registers sound amongst other things.

449 C
All the others will lead to one or more pupils dilating.

450 B
451 C
452 B
453 B
454 B
455 A
456 C
457 D
The others are signs, dizziness is a symptom.

458 C
The other 30% is found in bodily fluids such as blood and saliva.

459 C
17" = 44cm.

460 C
Because of peripheral vasodilation the skin should appear flushed and warm.

461 C
462 B
463 D
464 D
465 B
466 B
467 B
468 C
469 C
A lowered blood pressure usually accompanies a faint.

470 B
Although SIDS can happen at any time up to the age of 1 year.

471 C
You must remove the chemical as soon as possible to prevent further damage. Do not allow contaminated water to enter the good eye.

472 A
473 C
474 D
475 B
476 C
477 A
478 C
479 True
480 True
481 True
482 True
483 True
484 False
The uterine arteries are branches of the internal iliac artery.

485 True
486 True
487 True
488 True

489 True
490 True
491 False
492 False
Crowning is the appearance of the head.

493 True
494 True
495 True
496 True
497 True
498 True
499 False
Infections are very common with burns. Cover with a sterile dressing.

500 True
501 True
502 True
503 False
NEVER remove foreign objects from a wound. Apply pressure and sterile dressings AROUND the object.

504 True
505 True
506 True
If you cannot palpate a pulse distal to a fracture site it may be a sign of vascular impairment.

507 False
A sign is something you can see, a symptom is something the patient tells you.

508 False
The three factors used to make a patient assessment are history, signs and symptoms.

509 False
NEVER burst blisters - they protect the burn from infection.

510 False
YOUR safety comes first.

511 True
512 False
The first function in a primary survey is airway, followed by breathing and circulation.

513 False
The lungs are in the thoracic cavity.

514 False
Glands without ducts secrete hormones, glands with ducts secrete enzymes.

515 True
516 False
The spinal column contains 33 vertebrae which are irregular bones.

517 False
The cranium has 8 bones.

518 False
Lateral means away from the midline of the body.

519 True
520 True
521 True
Cardiac, skeletal and smooth.

522 True
523 True
524 True
525 False
The stomach contents are acidic.

526 True
527 True
528 False
Nausea is a typical sign of shock.

529 False
The skin has 2 layers, the dermis and epidermis.

530 True
531 True
532 True

533 True
534 False
Vitamin B12 is water soluble.

535 True
536 True
537 True
High blood pressure can lead to a blood vessel bursting in the brain.

538 True
539 True
540 True
541 True
542 True
543 False
544 True
545 True
546 False
Chickenpox is category 2 infectious disease.

547 False
548 True
549 True
550 True
551 False
Kinematics looks at the forces and mechanisms involved in an accident to work out possible injuries.

552 False
High blood sugar is hyperglycaemia, low is hypoglycaemia.

553 True
554 False
Dysphagia is difficulty in swallowing.

555 True
556 False
The stomach lies within the epigastric, umbilical and left hypochondrium regions.

557 True
558 True

559 False
One leg is equal to 18% of the body area with regard to the rule of nines.

560 False
One arm represents 9% of the body area in a child with regard to the rule of nines.

561 True
562 False
Abortion is the expulsion before the 24th week.

563 False
Neurogenic shock occurs when there is serious neurological impairment e.g. spinal cord injury. Hypovolaemic shock occurs with severe haemorrhage.

564 True
565 False
Asthma is a reversible obstruction caused by spasm of the smooth muscle due to irritation not infection.

566 True
567 False
Plasma is 55% of total blood volume, solids account for the other 45%.

568 False
Anthrax is a category 2 infectious disease.

569 True
570 False
Cavitation is caused by blunt or penetrating trauma.

571 False
Patients with circulatory or respiratory problems will almost always want to sit bolt upright since this eases breathing.

572 True
573 True

574 False
Confused scores 4 on the Glasgow Coma Scale.

575 True
576 False
The average length of the adult spinal cord is 16-18 inches.

577 False
The cerebrum is the largest part of the brain.

578 True
579 False
There are 31 pairs of spinal nerves.

580 False
Level of consciousness is determined after the ABC.

581 False
There are 4 stages to a grand mal seizure, aura, rigidity, convulsions and recovery.

582 False
Average stroke volume is 70ml.

583 False
The wall of the heart is made up of three layers, the endo-cardium (inner), the myocar-dium (middle) and the pericardium.

584 True
585 True
The bicuspid valve is on the left side of the heart and the tricuspid is on the right.

586 False
The left ventricle pumps blood to the rest of the body and the right ventricle pumps blood to the lungs.

587 True
588 True
589 True
590 True

591 False
Extensor response scores 2 on the Glasgow Coma Scale.

592 False
Pulmonary is associated with the lungs.

593 True
594 False
Leukocytes fight infection. Thrombocytes initiate the blood clotting procedure.

595 False
Erythrocytes number approximately 5.5 million per cubic millimetre of blood. Leukocytes number approximately 9,000 per cubic millimetre.

596 True
597 True
598 True
Apply pressure around the object to try and arrest the haemorrhage but do not remove the object or press directly on it.

599 False
A contusion is a bruise, an incision is caused by a sharp knife.

600 True
601 True
602 False
The pleura has two layers, the visceral pleura which attaches to the lungs and the parietal pleura which attaches to the inside of the thoracic cavity.

603 False
The left lung has only two lobes to accommodate the position of the heart.

604 False
Patients with chronic bronchitis should only be given low concentrations of oxygen, usually 28% or less, because of the likelihood of hypoxic drive being present.

605 True
Afferent neurones are sensory, efferent are motor.

606 True
607 True
608 True
609 True
610 True
Head injuries do not produce signs of shock.

611 False
DO NOT give oxygen to victims of paraquat poisoning as this only makes the problem worse. This situation is one of the VERY few in which oxygen should not be given.

612 False
Whooping cough is a category 1 infectious disease.

613 True
614 False
The cranial nerves are linked directly to the organ(s) they control.

615 True
616 True
617 True
618 True
Raising the legs and lowering the head prevents aspiration of stomach contents.

619 False
The pillow will cause hyperflexion of the neck. The head should be in neutral alignment.

620 True
The head injured patient is best placed in the recumbent position to maintain proper cerebral perfusion.

621 True
622 True
623 False
Ligaments attach bone to bone.

624 False
A strain is a tearing or wrenching of a muscle through overstretching.

625 True
The three physical chemical forms are solid, liquid and gas.

626 False
Entonox will leak into the pleural space quickly thereby making the problem worse.

627 False
Haemoglobin has an affinity for carbon monoxide. High levels of oxygenation are required in order to replace it.

628 True
629 False
Since there may be problems breathing, patients in status epilepticus should be given oxygen.

630 False
The lowest Glasgow Coma Score is 3.

631 False
In a contre-coup injury, the brain impacts on the opposite side of the skull creating an internal injury opposite to the external injury.

632 True

633 True
Intercranial haemorrhage compresses the optic nerve on the injured side causing the pupil to dilate.

634 True
635 False
636 False
Rabies is a category 3 infectious disease.

637 True
In an infant the ratio is slightly different and head and neck accounts for 18% of the total surface area.

638 False
The endometrium is the inner layer of the uterus, myometrium the middle layer and perimetrium the outer layer.

639 False
You should splint all fractures in some way to stop movement of the bone ends causing further damage.

640 False
The respiratory centre is situated in the medulla oblongata.

641 True
The left bronchus is narrower than the right because the left lung has only two lobes.

642 True
The lungs have their own blood and nervous supply and these enter the lungs through the hilum.

643 False
Hypoxia is a lack of oxygen to the tissues.

644 True
Impulses also pass this way to the intercostal muscles.

645 False
The stimulation for chronic bronchitics to breathe comes from the same chemo-receptors now measuring a decreased oxygen content in the blood instead of a raised carbon dioxide content.

646 True
647 False
Haemothorax is blood in the pleural cavity. Pneumothorax is air in the pleural cavity.

648 True
649 True
650 True
The tricuspid valve is on the right side of the heart and the bicuspid valve on the left.

651 False
Glasgow Coma Scores range from 3 (worst) to 15 (best).

652 False
Multipolar neurones are usually efferent.

653 False
Around 700 people die annually from burns.

654 False
One adult arm is 9% of the body area.

655 True
656 True
657 False
Partial thickness burns have 2 categories, superficial and deep.

658 False
Hyperglycaemia has a slow onset.

659 True
660 True
661 False
Do not induce vomiting in any poisoning incident.

662 True
663 False
There a 6 types of fracture, compound, simple, comminuted, greenstick, impacted and complicated.

664 False
Approximately 25% of the population will at some time experience some form of mental illness.

665 True
666 True
667 True
668 False
The cerebrum has 2 hemispheres.

669 True
670 True
671 True
672 False
Periosteum is the covering for bones. The peritoneum is a protective layer in the abdomen.

673 False
There are 14 facial bones and 8 cranial bones.

674 False
The zygoma and zygomatic arch form part of the facial skeleton (they are commonly called the cheek bones).

675 False
676 False
677 True
678 False
Inspired air contains 20% oxygen, expired contains 16%.

679 False
Acquired Immune Deficiency Syndrome.

680 True

681 False
Treat an undiagnosed fracture as a fracture until proven otherwise.

682 True
683 True
684 False
Leukocytes fight infection. Platelets form part of the clotting process.

685 True
686 True
687 True
688 False
Venous blood has given up its oxygen and will therefore be dark red. It does not have the pressure of arterial blood and will therefore ooze rather than gush from the wound.

689 False
Hypovolaemic shock displays a rapid, shallow pulse.

690 True
691 True
692 True
693 True
694 True
695 False
The meninges surround the brain and spinal cord.

696 True
The four principle parts of the brain are the cerebrum, cerebellum, mid brian and diencephalon.

697 False
A fitting epileptic patient should be protected from injury without restraint.

698 True
699 False
There are 31 pairs of spinal nerves.

700 True

701 False
Although airway maintenance is the priority the spine should be kept in neutral alignment.

702 True
703 False
You should never test for crepitus as it is very painful and further fragments the ends of the bone.

704 False
While tourniquets stop the blood from exiting the wound they also deprive the distal tissues of oxygenated blood and should therefore not be used.

705 True
706 True
707 True
708 True
709 True
710 True
711 True
712 False
Bone is 20% water, 30-40% organic material and 40-50% inorganic material.

713 True
714 False
The femur is a long bone. An example of a flat bone is the maxilla.

715 False
A petit mal is a period of vagueness. A grand mal has four stages.

716 True
717 True
718 False
Internal respiration takes place at tissue level, external respiration takes place at the lungs.

719 False
The cerebrum controls voluntary muscle movement and the cerebellum controls involuntary muscle movement such as the diaphragm.

720 True
Haversian canals are microscopic canals in mature compact bone which accommodate blood vessels and nerves.

721 True
722 True
The skin can alter body temperature by use of the sweat glands and alteration of blood supply to its surface.

723 False
A gliding joint allows free movement in two planes only, left to right and back to front.

724 False
2 man CPR has the ratio of 5 compressions to 1 inflation.

725 False
There is still clear passage around the oropharyngeal airway for vomit to enter the lungs.

726 False
An asphyxiated patient requires 100% oxygen therapy.

727 False
External respiration takes place in the lungs, internal respiration at the tissues.

728 True
729 True
While the smallest structure within the lung is the alveolus, the smallest division is that of each lobe into lobules. Each lobule is self sufficient having its own blood and nerve supply.

730 True
731 False
Greenstick fractures only occur in children due to the flexibility of their bones.

732 False
The epiglottis lies over the larynx.

733 False
The air is moistened as it is taken into the body.

734 True
735 False
While the organs of respiration are in the chest, the centre which controls them is in the medulla.

736 False
Cardiac arrest means an absence of a pulse.

737 True
738 False
739 False
Chemoreceptors are sensitive to the levels of carbon dioxide in the blood.

740 True
741 False
The periosteum is profusely supplied with blood and lymph vessels and nerves.

742 False
Average tidal volume is 500ml.

743 False
There are 14 facial bones.

744 False
By reducing the traction the bones will meet again causing pain and increase the possibility of entrapment of blood vessels or nerves.

745 True
746 True

747 False
Check both distal and proximal to ensure circulation below the injury.

748 False
Open fractures are associated with external wounds.

749 True
750 False
A ball and socket joint allows for movement in all directions. The shoulder and the hip are examples.

751 False
The larynx is respiratory only.

752 False
The left lung has 2 lobes, the right lung has 3.

753 True
754 True
755 True
756 True
757 False
Right sided heart failure is usually secondary to left.

758 True
759 False
Unconscious CVA patients should be nursed paralysed side up to ensure adequate neurovascular supply to the affected side.

760 False
A faint is syncope, a CVA is apoplexy.

761 False
Haemodialysis patients are prone to hypotension.

762 False
In normal labour the first stage takes the longest.

763 False
764 False
In a premature baby the skull may appear unduly large.

765 False
Wrap the cord in warm, moist sterile dressings and promptly transport the mother in the recovery position with the head down.

766 True
767 False
Superficial burns do cause redness and blistering but are not deep enough to cause nerve damage.

768 False
Entonox cylinders are blue with a blue and white segmented neck.

769 False
1 hand = 1% of the body area with regard to the rule of nines.

770 True
Cardiogenic shock results from some heart conditions.

771 False
Ischaemia is due to a progressive narrowing of coronary arteries and is therefore a chronic condition.

772 False
Patients with congestive cardiac failure should travel sitting upright but more often than not the patient will dictate how they want to sit.

773 True
Anaphylactic shock may result from an insect sting (injected substance).

774 True
Spinal injury could lead to neurogenic shock.

775 True
776 False
777 False
Axons transmit impulses away from the cell body.

778 True

779 False
Lie in the medulla.

780 True
781 True
782 False
Burns from boiling water and fat cool slowly causing more skin damage. Cool the area immediately.

783 False
The small intestine is approximately 5 metres long.

784 True
785 False
Do not insert anything into the mouth any further than you can see.

786 False
Folding flexible catheters may kink them, reducing their diameter and rendering them useless.

787 True
788 True
Carbon monoxide or cyanide poisoning can lead to asphyxia.

789 False
Over-oxygenation can cause blindness. If the neonate requires oxygenation use an oxygen funnel to create an oxygen enriched atmosphere close to the face.

790 False
External respiration takes place in the lungs, internal respiration at the tissues.

791 False
Entonox is 50% oxygen and 50% nitrous oxide.

792 True
Carbon dioxide increases the acidity of the blood. The pH scale has acids at a lower number than alkalines.

793 True

794 False

At least two members of a crew are required to remove a crash helmet.

795 False

Angina is caused by a build up of fatty deposits in coronary arteries and is therefore chronic.

796 True

797 False

Shock is a clinical condition requiring proper treatment. Warm tea may make the patient feel sick and hinder further procedures.

798 True

799 True

800 False

801 True

A silent myocardial infarction will not exhibit the symptom of chest pain.

802 True

803 False

The 4 pulmonary veins carry blood from the lungs to the heart.

804 True

805 False

An incision is made by a sharp edge, a laceration is a tearing of the tissues.

806 True

807 False

Oropharyngeal airways do not guarantee a patent airway, only prevent the tongue from occluding it.

808 False

A sprain is a tearing or wrenching of a ligament at a joint. A strain is a tearing or wrenching of a muscle.

809 True

810 Arteriosclerosis

811 Aneurysm

812 Amnesia

813 Aspirator

814 Antipsychotic

815 Anoxia

816 Apnoea

817 Ankle

818 Axilla

819 Auscultation

820 Bile

821 Breech

822 Brain

823 Bends

824 Bilateral

825 Bicuspid

826 Bradycardia

827 Bronchitis

828 Brachial

829 Bladder

830 Capillaries

831 Cerebrospinal fluid (CSF)

832 Cyanosis

833 Colles

834 Carotid

835 Cerebellum

836 Cardiovascular

837 Cerebrovascular accident (CVA)

838 Cardiac

839 Caecum

840 Dehydration

841 Diabetes

842 Drowsiness

843 Depression

844 Distal

845 Dyspnoea

846 Diaphragm

847 Diaphoresis

848 Diastole

849 Embolism / Embolus

850 Emphysema

851 Ectopic

852 Epistaxis

853 Eclampsia

854 Emergency

855 Effusion

856 Endocardium

857 Embryo

858 Fatigue

859 Fibrillation

860 Foxtrot

861 Fainting

862 Febrile convulsion

863 Femoral

864 Femur

865 Facial

866 Fowler

867 Fallopian

868 Foetus

869 Faeces

870 Geriatrics

871 Glaucoma

872 Gland

873 Gene

874 Glucagon/ Glucose

875 Gastroenteritis

876 Glosso-phryngeal

877 Gestation

878 Gall bladder

879 Gangrene

880 Haematoma

881 Haemophilia

882 Humerus

883 Haemolysis

884 Haemorrhage

885 Haemoptysis

886 Haematemesis

887 Haemoglobin

888 Haematuria

889 Haemodialysis

890 Hypovolaemic
891 Haematology
892 Insulin
893 Infant
894 Inflammation
895 Incubator
896 Infarction
897 Ileum
898 Infertility
899 Immune
900 Immobilisation
901 Incontinence
902 Jagged
903 Jaundice
904 Jugular
905 Joule
906 Joint
907 Jejunum
908 Jaw
909 Ketoacidosis (Ketosis)
910 Kidney
911 Kneecap
912 Kyphosis
913 Kussmauls
914 Kinetics
915 Laparoscopy
916 Laceration
917 Ligament
918 Lactic Acid
919 Leukocyte
920 Legs
921 Larynx
922 Laryngitis
923 Lateral
924 Meninges
925 Mast
926 Medial
927 Melaena
928 Maxilla
929 Monoplegia
930 Mandible
931 Myocardium
932 Mastication
933 Mediastinum
934 Nebuliser
935 Neurogenic
936 Neonate
937 Narcosis
938 Nephritis
939 Necrosis
940 Neck
941 Nephron
942 Nasopharynx
943 Nausea
944 Nervous
945 Obstetrics
946 Opium
947 Oedema
948 Orthopaedics
949 Olfactory
950 Oesophagus
951 Osmosis
952 Oculomotor
953 Pandemic
954 Paraquat
955 Pain
956 Pallor
957 Palpitation
958 Pacemaker
959 Paediatrics
960 Para-sympathetic
961 Paraplegia
962 Pancreas
963 Regurgitation
964 Rubella
965 Rib
966 Retina
967 Radiation
968 Renal
969 Referred
970 Recovery
971 Relapse
972 Salbutamol
973 Scald
974 Shock
975 Septum
976 Sprain
977 Scapula
978 Schizophrenia
979 Sciatic
980 Spleen
981 Systole
982 Thrombus
983 Tuberculosis
984 Temazepam
985 Tachycardia
986 Tachypnoea
987 Temporal
988 Tetraplegia
989 Trachea
990 Tamponade
991 Tibia
992 Thorax
993 Urticaria
994 Urinary
995 Ulna
996 Umbilical
997 Urethra
998 Whiplash
999 Wheeze
1000 Warfarin

NOTES